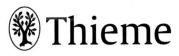

Contact Lens Complications

Etiology, Pathogenesis, Prevention, Therapy

Hans-Walter Roth, M.D.

Director
Institute of Contact Lens Optics
Ulm, Germany

476 illustrations
38 tables

Thieme
Stuttgart · New York

Library of Congress-in-Publication Data is available from the publisher

This book is an authorized translation of the German edition published and copyrighted 2002 by Georg Thieme Verlag, Stuttgart, Germany. Title of the German edition: Kontaktlinsenkomplikationen, Ätiologie, Pathogenese, Prophylaxe, Therapie.

Translated by
Donald L. MacKeen, M.S., Ph.D., Bethesda MD, USA
and Ethan Taub, M.D., Zurich, Switzerland.

© 2003 Georg Thieme Verlag,
Rüdigerstrasse 14, 70469 Stuttgart, Germany
http://www.thieme.de
Thieme New York, 333 Seventh Avenue,
New York, NY 10001 USA
http://www.thieme.com

Typesetting by Druckhaus Götz, 71636 Ludwigsburg
Printed in Germany by Appl, Wemding

ISBN 3-13-127791-2 (GTV)
ISBN 1-58890-132-7 (TNY)   1 2 3 4 5

Foreword

Contact lenses are currently used electively by 80 to 100 million patients worldwide to correct refractive errors of vision. With so many patients at increasing risk for device-related ocular complications, Dr. Roth's excellent treatise, *Contact Lens Complications*, is a timely and important work. Long familiar and available to European readers in German, the current translation and publication of an English edition is a most welcome development for all practitioners and academics who practice both the scientific and clinical art of contactology throughout the world. The timing of publication of this superb monograph is particularly fortunate because it coincides with the introduction into clinical practice of a new generation of contact lenses: hyper oxygen-transmissible contact lenses recently approved for up to 30-night extended wear by the Food and Drug Administration, USA. Thus, it is more important than ever for con-

tactology practitioners to be familiar with contact-lens–induced eye problems.

Outstanding features of the text are brevity without sacrificing comprehensiveness or clarity, and excellent color photographs. These features will ensure instant popularity of the English edition among both a generation of optometric students and ophthalmology residents. Indeed, it appears that an old classic has been reborn for the world community at large.

H. Dwight Cavanagh, M.D., Ph.D., F.A.C.S.
Professor and Vice-Chairman
The Dr. W. Maxwell Thomas Chair in Ophthalmology
Associate Dean for Clinical Services
and Medical Director
Zale Lipshy University Hospital, TX, USA

Preface

Contact lenses are unquestionably a useful aid in the treatment of refractive problems and of many diseases of the eye. They can be used to compensate for optical errors or as an ocular bandage, protective covering, or drug delivery system. They improve the wearer's appearance and expand the field of vision; they perform the function of a destroyed cornea or cover an iris that has been damaged by trauma or disease. They facilitate many sporting activities and indeed open certain professions to persons with impaired vision who would not otherwise be able to pursue them.

Yet contact lenses also have disadvantages. They exert chronic pressure on the anterior surface of the eye, disturb the convection of tears, and impair immune responses in the eye through chronic foreign-body irritation, thus potentially causing complications in the anterior ocular segment. Finally, contact lenses can mask certain types of primary ocular illness, which, in the setting of contact lens wear, may be difficult to diagnose.

Like any effective medical treatment, contact lenses have not only a therapeutic effect, but also undesirable side effects. A wide variety of contact lens complications have been reported in recent years, most of which require treatment by an ophthalmologist. Contact lens complications are sometimes easily mistaken for other ocular diseases, and vice versa; the diagnostic evaluation of contact lens complications thus requires considerable expertise on the ophthalmologist's part.

A cursory glance at this book reveals that the ocular complications of contact lenses are numerous and varied, and may create the impression that the risk of wearing them is incalculably high. Yet this is certainly not the case. The multiplicity of complications in no way diminishes the therapeutic value of contact lenses, as the actual frequency of complications, according to many well-performed, international, longitudinal studies, is well below 1%—a rate that is hardly matched by many other forms of routine treatment in ophthalmology. Safety is assured by proper lens care and handling on the part of the patient, and by frequent and thorough follow-up examinations on the part of the ophthalmologist.

This book is meant to be useful to everyone involved in contactology, including resident physicians and ophthalmologists who have just started fitting contact lenses. We have avoided extensive discussions of basic science that can be found in other texts and have tried to use terminology that will be transparent even to persons with little experience in contactology. Examining techniques and findings are presented in such a way that they could be duplicated by any ophthalmologist, whether in an academic institution or in private practice.

In writing this book, the author has had to face certain inevitable difficulties. This is the first comprehensive publication in ophthalmology addressing the more important complications of contact lenses, and the causes and interrelationships of many of the findings discussed here are still imperfectly understood. Furthermore, contact lenses have not been in use long enough to allow a complete assessment of their long-term complications. This will have to await future publications by other investigators.

This book is the fruit of more than 25 years of research and teaching in applied contact optics in the University Ophthalmology Department and Army Hospital in Ulm, Germany, at the Institute for Contact Optics in Ulm, and at the Center for Sight, Georgetown University Medical Center, Washington, DC.

I would like to thank my teachers in contactology, Drs R Marquardt in Ulm, W Erich in Homburg/Saar, the late H Kemmetmueller in Vienna, the late P Halberg in New York, M Lemp and D MacKeen in Washington, and the late Jonathan Kersley in London. I would also like to thank the numerous others who taught me through their published works, and, finally, the staff of Georg Thieme Verlag for their invaluable assistance in producing this book.

Washington DC–Ulm/Danube, Spring 2003

Hans-Walter Roth

Contents

1 Problems Caused by Contact Lenses 1

Overview 2
Materials and Manufacture 3
Fitting Technique 3
Contraindications 4
Hygiene 4
Loss of Contact Lenses 4

Ocular Trauma 5
Maximum Wearing Time 5
Patients with Systemic Diseases 5
Patients at High Risk of Complications 6
Psychological Factors 6
Summary: The Risk of Injury 6

2 Patient Counseling and Examination 7

Patient Counseling 8
History Taking 9
Examination 10
General 10
Lid 10
Conjunctiva 11
Cornea 14
Inner Eye 21

Intraocular Pressure 21
Refractive Error and Visual Acuity 21
Binocular Vision 21
Inspection of Contact Lenses 21
Inspection of Contact Lens Cases 22
Documentation of Findings 23
Follow-up 24

3 Pathologic Findings 25

Lid 26
Anatomy and Physiology 26
Increased Lid Tension and Blepharospasm .. 26
Ptosis 27
Lid Swelling and Edema 27
Infectious Blepharitis, Squamous Blepharitis,
Ulceration 29
Lid Injury 34
Conjunctiva 35
Anatomy and Physiology 35
Tarsal Conjunctiva 35
Follicular Swelling, Papillary Hypertrophy,
Giant Papillary Conjunctivitis 35
Bulbar Conjunctiva 40
Conjunctival Edema and Acute Chemosis . 40
Subconjunctival Hemorrhage 42
Focal Conjunctival Hyperemia 52
Sclera 58
Anatomy and Physiology 58
Pathology 58
Vasodilatation and Inflammation 58
Injury and Hemorrhage 58
Cornea 59
Anatomy and Physiology 59
Epithelial Changes 59
Edema and Staining 60
Stippling 60
Streaks and Spiral Traces 62
Indentations 62
Cracks 62

Spiders 62
Mosaics 62
Nummules and Pseudoinfiltrates 64
Corneal Erosions 66
Bizarre Epithelial Defects, Branched
Defects, Pseudoherpetic Defects 71
Bubble Formation and Pseudokeratitis
Bullosa 75
Stromal Changes 75
Edema 75
Tight Lens Syndrome 78
Toxic Keratopathy 80
Mixed Solution Syndrome 88
Corneal Deprivation Syndrome 90
Post-Heat Syndrome 92
Vascularization 92
Infection 99
Clouding and Scars 105
Changes of Descemet's Membrane and the
Endothelium 109
Changes of Descemet's Membrane 109
Endothelial Changes 109
Topographic Changes 109
Contour Changes 110
Pachymetric Changes 114
Inner Eye 116
Iritis, Uveitis, Panophthalmitis 116
Cataract 117
Intraocular Hypertension, Glaucoma 117
Retinal Diseases and Detachment 117

4 Visual Impairment 119

Visual Impairment 120
Causes of Visual Impairment 121
 Changes in Refraction 121
  Faulty Lens Handling and Insertion, Lens
  Loss 121
 Permanent Visual Impairment 121
  Primary Ocular Diseases Masked by
  Contact Lenses 121
  Material Defects and Defective Lenses 123
 Intermittent Visual Impairment 123

Fitting Errors 123
Orthokeratological Side Effects 125
Spectacle-Blur Phenomenon and Corneal
Distortion Syndrome 125
 Wetting Problems 125
Glare 127
 Causes of Glare 127
Diagnostic Evaluation of Visual Impairment
and Glare 128

5 Causes of Contact Lens Damage 129

Handling, Hygiene, Wearing Times 130
 The Patient's Hands 130
 The Lens Case 130

Wearing Times 132
Fitting Errors 132

6 Alterations of Contact Lenses 137

Wetting Problems 138
Material Defects 139
Discoloration and Fading 145

Deposits 147
 Components of Tear Fluid 151
 Jelly Bumps 151

7 Primary Fitting and Wearing Problems 159

Systemic Disease 160
 Febrile Illnesses, Immune Compromise,
 Medication Use 160
 Allergy 160
Primary Ocular Disease 161
 Lid Diseases 161
 Conjunctival Diseases 165

Corneal Diseases 171
Tear Deficiency, Disorders of Lacrimation,
Dry Eye 171
 Pathophysiology 171
 Clinical Course 173
 Clinical Testing 183
Other Eye Diseases 184

8 Eye Injuries in Contact Lens Wearers 185

Types of Ocular Trauma 186
 Trauma Involving Foreign Bodies 186
 Perforated Globe 186

Ocular Contusion 186
Chemical Injury 187
Consequences for Contact Lens Wearers 188

9 Frequency of Contact Lens Complications 189

Analysis of Contact Lens Complications 190

10 Treatment of Contact Lens Complications 193

General Aspects 194
General Treatment Procedures 195
Special Treatment Procedures 196
 Lid Diseases 196
  Blepharospasm 196
  Ptosis 196

Lid Edema 196
Squamous Blepharitis 196
Lid Trauma 196
Conjunctival Diseases 197
 Giant Papillary Conjunctivitis 197
 Conjunctival Chemosis 197

Conjunctival Hemorrhage 197
Conjunctival Trauma 197
Nonspecific Conjunctival Hyperemia 198
Bacterial Conjunctivitis 198
Viral Conjunctivitis 198
Fungal Conjunctivitis 198
Scleral Diseases 198
Corneal Diseases 198
Corneal Edema 198
Corneal Erosion 198
Bullous Keratopathy 199
Tight Lens Syndrome 199
Toxic Keratopathy 199
Corneal Deprivation Syndrome 199

Post-Heat Syndrome 199
Keratitis, Corneal Infiltrates, Corneal
Ulcers 199
Corneal Vascularization 200
Corneal Scars 200
Corneal Deformation 200
Folds in Descemet's Membrane,
Endothelial Changes 200
Intraocular Findings 200
Glaucoma 200
Dry Eye, Tear Deficiency Syndrome 201
Accidents, Mechanical Trauma, Chemical
Trauma 202

References 203

Index to Text 209

Index to Illustrations 212

1 Problems Caused by Contact Lenses

Overview

Materials and Manufacture

Fitting Technique

Contraindications

Hygiene

Loss of Contact Lenses

Ocular Trauma

Maximum Wearing Time

Patients with Systemic Diseases

Patients at High Risk of Complications

Psychological Factors

Summary: The Risk of Injury

Overview

A contact lens is a rigid optical device that maintains close, prolonged contact with the living tissue of the eye. Contact lenses can be worn for many years without difficulty, but only if they are made of a well-chosen material, correctly shaped, and properly fitted. Complications can be prevented by precise fitting and regular follow-up by an ophthalmologist experienced in the recognition and management of the associated pathological conditions. The universally acknowledged importance of contact lenses in contemporary ophthalmology does not obviate the need for careful weighing of indications and contraindications (Tables **1** and **2**), advantages and disadvantages (Tables **3** and **4**), and risks and benefits, as with any other form of medical treatment.

Contact lenses are a valuable aid to vision in the presence of severe refractive errors, and an irreplaceable component of treatment for certain chronic diseases of the eye. Yet their use is not without risk. Like any other form of medical treatment, they have both desired and undesired effects. Some wearers of contact lenses will develop ocular complications, ranging from harmless irritation of the lids or conjunctiva to sight-threatening corneal ulceration. In a few reported cases, eyes have even been lost through the wearing of contact lenses. Fortunately, these disasters are extremely rare, but they serve to remind us of the dangers against which we must be on guard.

Table **1**   Indications for contact lenses
Cosmetic reasons
Myopia
Hypermetropia
Regular or irregular astigmatism
Anisometropia, aniseikonia
Corneal scars
Aphakia
Post-keratoplasty
Occupation or athletic activities
Iris lesion, pupillary dysfunction
Bandage lens
Drug-delivery vehicle
Particular diseases of the anterior segment

Table **2**   Contraindications of contact lenses
Chronic irritation of the lids, conjunctiva, or cornea
Malformation of the anterior segment
Absence of lacrimation
Inability to comply with lens hygiene regimen
Difficulty in handling lenses
Long-term use of ocular medications

Table **3**   Advantages of contact lenses over spectacles
Near invisibility
Improvement of vision in high ametropia
Improvement of vision in irregular astigmatism
Equal image size for patients with different refractive errors in the two eyes
Containment effect in keratoconus and progressive myopia
Bandage effect in chronic ocular diseases
Medication vehicle for long-term delivery

Table **4**   Disadvantages of contact lenses compared with spectacles
Need for conscientious lens care
Limited wearing time
Greater risk of injury
Easier to lose, harder to find
Risk of infection
Risk of allergic reaction
Greater difficulty in handling
More frequent ophthalmological follow-up necessary
Shorter life of lenses
Limited durability
Metabolic and mechanical disturbance of the eye
Possible psychological disturbance
Need for thorough patient education

Materials and Manufacture

Contact lenses are apt to cause complications because they pose a constant challenge to the normal functioning and immune defenses of the anterior segment of the eye. Their adverse mechanical effects may include deformation of the corneal curvature and thinning of the corneal stroma due to chronic pressure upon it. By disturbing corneal metabolism, they may induce swelling of the corneal stroma and alter the structure and cellular composition of the endothelium. They also raise the temperature of the lids, conjunctiva, and cornea by a few degrees Celsius, and thereby promote inflammation.

The manufacture of contact lenses thus demands not only high mechanical precision in the shaping of the lens, but also a lens material that is transparent, chemically pure, durable, nontoxic, and nonallergenic. These requirements are not easy to meet.

A further difficulty is that nearly all errors in fitting, choice of lens material, or disinfecting technique do not become manifest when the patient begins to wear the lens, but only later, through the pathological changes they produce in the eye. Thus, a careful prefitting history and examination, close supervision of the wearer, and regular follow-up are essential for the prevention of later problems.

There are innumerable reports of contact lens complications due to improper fitting, careless follow-up, lack of adherence to the guidelines for lens hygiene, and wearing the lenses for longer than the recommended time. Such complications are the principal difference between spectacles and contact lenses. Spectacles make prolonged contact only with the skin and thus cause, at worst, skin irritation, while contact lenses make prolonged contact with sensitive, metabolically active epithelial cells bathed in a bodily fluid (tears), and can easily damage them. The risk of complications is immediately clear when contact lenses are properly regarded as a type of synthetic medical implant, comparable to other devices such as artificial hips, synthetic vascular grafts, silicone breast implants, and artificial heart valves.

Many problems result from the interaction of synthetic materials with tissue, the most common of which is giant papillary conjunctivitis (GPC). A perfectly nonallergenic, hapten-free material for contact lenses has yet to be developed.

Fitting Technique

The chronic pressure exerted by a contact lens on the anterior surface of the eye can be kept to a minimum by the exact fitting of a lens with an aspheric inner surface, but will nevertheless, in most cases, cause topographical changes of the cornea after prolonged wearing. The continual changes in corneal thickness and contour over the course of a day, and over the years, cannot easily be summarized by a mathematical formula. There will never be an ideal contact lens that always lies exactly parallel to the corneal surface at every point, exerting a constant and spatially unvarying pressure on it, yet also—as the physiologists demand—gliding freely over it with every blink. Optimal fitting thus represents a compromise between an even distribution of pressure and a minimal disturbance of corneal metabolism. Poor fitting may lead to corneal damage, such as irregular astigmatism or Type C keratoconus.

Contraindications

Contact lenses are contraindicated by all acute and chronic processes affecting the anterior segment of the eye. For example, squamous blepharitis, chronic conjunctivitis, recurring keratitis, hordeola, and chalazia may all recur or worsen acutely when contact lenses are worn. Growths on the corneal or conjunctival surface, such as pinguecula or pterygia, contraindicate the wearing of certain kinds of lenses. Many conditions affecting the endothelium are also contraindications; patients with endothelial dystrophy should not wear contact lenses for cosmesis. Nor should contact lenses be worn in the presence of a filtering bleb after the surgical creation of a fistula.

Patients who must regularly use eye drops for the treatment of glaucoma or other disorders are only rarely suitable candidates for contact lenses. Lens wearing alters the pharmacokinetics of instilled agents and may necessitate a change of the dosage.

Contact lenses must sit on a cushion of tear fluid to be able to glide freely over the corneal surface. Soft lenses need a small additional amount of tear fluid to stay elastic. Therefore, each contact lens, depending on its type, composition, and mode of wearing, requires up to 1 ml of tear fluid daily, a quantity equaling the entire daily production of tears in a healthy eye. Disorders of lacrimation thus predispose to contact lens complications. Artificial tears may compensate temporarily for diminished lacrimation but must not be used as a permanent measure, because, by eliminating the reflex drive to lacrimation, they diminish it further. The preservatives found in moisturizing eye drops may also damage the eye with prolonged use.

Hygiene

All contact lenses, whether conventional, disposable, or for extended wear, should be regularly removed for cleaning and disinfection. Among the many different disinfecting and cleaning solutions now available, some may irritate or injure eyes that are sensitive to particular components of their formulation. Allergic reactions are seen much less frequently with the newer types of solution, but there is still a danger of severe toxic keratopathy, particularly when incompatible solutions are mixed.

Loss of Contact Lenses

Contact lenses are easier to lose than spectacles, and much harder to find. A surefire way to lose contact lenses is to wear them while swimming, diving, or surfing. Sudden jerking of the head, as when it is struck in a boxing match or brawl, can also easily dislodge contact lenses. Such events sometimes have medicolegal consequences.

Sports involving sudden, massive bodily movements, such as horseback riding or sky diving, necessitate lenses of larger than usual diameter, but such lenses cannot be worn as long as ordinary lenses. Thus, persons engaging in such sports should also have a pair of ordinary lenses for normal wear.

Ocular Trauma

All contact lenses cause a certain amount of epithelial microtrauma during normal wear. The corneal and conjunctival surfaces may be injured when the lens is inserted or removed, and may even be cut if the lens is defective. In such cases, lens wearing is discontinued and the wound generally heals within a few days, though the potential for infection or ulceration exists.

Maximum Wearing Time

No type of contact lens can be worn indefinitely, and only a few types can be worn during sleep. The recommended maximum wearing time depends on the age of the lens and the amount of surface deposition. Changing disposable lenses in a weekly rhythm is a safe practice only if new lenses are used every week. Perhaps surprisingly, soft contact lenses developed for extended wear cause the most complications; when they are worn without interruption, the rate of complications rises exponentially with the duration of wear. Corneal ulcers are more than 30 times as common when contact lenses are worn for extended periods than when they are worn for no more than 18 hours a day.

Patients with Systemic Diseases

Most of the reported severe complications of contact lenses involve infection with *Pseudomonas* or *Acanthamoeba* infection. Corneal ulceration is usually caused by poor hygiene and excessively prolonged wear.

Diabetic patients are more likely to develop fungal infections, while immunocompromised patients, such as those with leukemia or AIDS and patients undergoing antineoplastic chemotherapy, are more likely to develop bacterial ulcers. The high risk of ocular infection in these groups of patients contraindicates the wearing of contact lenses.

Because many orally or parenterally administered medications, and their metabolic products, are secreted into the lacrimal fluid, the use of such medications contraindicates the wearing of hydrophilic or water-absorbing contact lenses. For example, in a patient taking oral calcium supplements, soft contact lenses of high water content may be irreversibly damaged within a few hours by deposition of insoluble calcium salts and proteins on their surface.

Many systemic diseases, including rheumatic diseases, thyroid and renal dysfunction, and other diseases treated with hormone supplementation, can alter the secretion of tears and thereby interfere with the wearing of contact lenses. The same is true of oral contraceptive use. The impairment of lacrimation may be asymptomatic until the patient begins wearing contact lenses.

Patients at High Risk of Complications

Contact lens fitting is not just a matter of measuring the refractive error and the corneal radius and diameter, calculating the desired lens parameters, and choosing the lenses accordingly. Rather, it requires a thorough knowledge of the anatomy and physiology of the living eye. For example, there is no textbook method for fitting contact lenses in an aphakic neonate. In such difficult cases, the ophthalmologist and contact lens team may need to call on many years of accumulated expertise.

Patients with keratoconus are also at high risk of complications. If the lens that is fitted is too flat, acute decompensation of the cone may occur practically overnight, leading to perforation and the need for immediate keratoplasty. An uneven distribution of pressure from the edge of the lens on the peripheral zone of the cornea may injure the epithelium. In patients with Type B keratoconus, the severe reduction of tear flow usually makes wearing lenses very difficult.

Older aphakic patients, too, are prone to complications of various types. Frequent lens loss and difficulties in handling limit the potential for successful contact lens wear in these patients. Lens fitting is especially difficult in this group after perforating injury or invasive ocular surgery. The resultant irregular astigmatism tends to make contact lenses unstable. Successful fitting requires both longstanding expertise and a sound biophysical understanding of the effect of lens pressure and the consequent corneal molding on a lacerated or scarred cornea.

Psychological Factors

Some patients are psychologically ill equipped to wear contact lenses. It is often advisable to recommend against wearing contact lenses for psychological reasons, even if the patient explicitly desires to wear them. The contact lens specialist should be able to recognize the potential for self-destructive and suicidal behavior, particularly in young, female patients with relationship difficulties, and should be ready to refer such patients for psychiatric help if necessary. A problem of another kind occurred in one of our patients, who complained of severe pain and visual disturbances while wearing contact lenses, although the ocular findings were normal. It turned out that her mother had forced her to wear contact lenses against her wishes. The ocular symptoms resolved when, on the doctor's orders, she stopped wearing the lenses.

Summary: The Risk of Injury

As we have seen, any contact lens may cause complications, potentially as severe as the loss of an eye. The most important preventive measures are a preliminary assessment and repeated follow-up by an ophthalmologist, and fitting by an experienced lens fitter. The patient must be made aware of the need to consult the ophthalmologist immediately for any problem that may arise. Only an explicit instruction to this effect can counteract the false impression of safety created by mass marketing, disposable lenses, internet advertising, and discount selling practices. As many years of clinical research have shown, contact lenses are not an optical product to be obtained by mail order or in the bargain basement. Only an experienced fitter can realize their potential as a valuable form of treatment for visual impairment and other ocular disorders.

2 Patient Counseling and Examination

Patient Counseling

History Taking

Examination

General

Lid

Conjunctiva

Cornea

Inner Eye

Intraocular Pressure

Refractive Error and Visual Acuity

Binocular Vision

Inspection of Contact Lenses

Inspection of Contact Lens Cases

Documentation of Findings

Follow-up

Patient Counseling

All patients need thorough counseling and instruction before they choose the type of contact lenses they will wear and as they begin to wear them. The major issues to be addressed are listed in Table **5**. The choice of contact lens is not simply a matter of finding the type that gives the best cosmetic result, as patients may at first assume, but requires consideration of patient-specific risks and other factors, particularly the patient's living and working environment. Despite recent advances in soft-lens technology, hard lenses are still better tolerated over the long term, though hydrophilic lenses may be better suited to the patient's lifestyle and desired manner of wearing. For patients who plan to wear contact lenses only occasionally, soft lenses are preferable; those who plan to wear contact lenses instead of spectacles over the long term are better served with hard lenses. Patients should be informed, however, that switching from hard contact lenses back to spectacles may be difficult. Long-term wearing of hard contact lenses can cause irregular astigmatism, leading to diminished visual acuity and increased glare; this is the so-called spectacle blur phenomenon. It often takes several months after the cessation of contact lens wear for these symptoms to resolve so that vision with spectacles is as good as before.

Lens care products are to be regarded as medications, and due attention should be paid to their storage, stability, and expiration dates. Every contact lens wearer should be adequately instructed about their use, effects, and potential complications. The proper choice of lens care system depends not only on the type of lens, but also on the type and rate of deposition on the lens surface, which varies from patient to patient. Those for whom lens care is difficult, such as patients with arthritis, should use only one cleaning agent, if possible. Those with particularly sensitive eyes should use hydrogen peroxide. Careful consideration should be given to the possible use of an additional cleaning solution, or of enzyme tablets.

The ever-decreasing cost of contact lenses and the introduction of disposable lenses have misled many wearers to imagine that contact lens optics is a routine matter, and that their purchase and use are a retail business like any other. Yet the fitting of contact lenses actually demands the highest expertise of the ophthalmologist and optician. Additionally, their physical specification and manufacture are an intricate technical process, at whose end the lenses can be safely handed over to the patient only when all of the problems discussed above have been resolved, unnecessary risks avoided, and possible contraindications ruled out. Finally, the prescriber of contact lenses must be certain that the patient can care for them properly and knows the problems that may arise with improper use.

Table **5**   Patient education
General reasons for wearing contact lenses
Pros and cons of contact lenses *vs.* spectacles
Problems in switching between contact lenses and spectacles
Problems in the workplace
Limited wearing time
Lens handling, insertion, removal
Lens cleaning
Lens disinfection
Frequency of replacement of short-term lenses
Contact lenses and use of medication
Contact lenses in patients with chronic illnesses
Follow-up examinations by the fitter or ophthalmologist
What to do in an emergency

History Taking

The patient's past medical history and review of systems may indicate the presence of an acute or chronic illness that would increase the risk of wearing contact lenses. Such illnesses, a history of major trauma, and the chronic use of medications of certain types may contraindicate wear. The use of oral contraceptives, pregnancy, and breastfeeding are also limiting factors. The patient should be asked about prior ocular injuries, infections, other diseases, and the prior use of eye drops.

If the data are available, the physician should also note any changes over time of the patient's spectacle prescription, which may indicate a progression of the refractive error. Finally, the patient should be asked whether contact lenses were previously prescribed or worn, with what result, and why a previous fitting was unsuccessful, if this was the case.

Examination

General

The tasks of the ophthalmologist include ocular examination before contact lens fitting, monitoring for potential problems in the initial adaptation phase, and regular follow-up thereafter. The routine ophthalmological examination of the contact lens wearer is the same as that of any other patient; its most important elements are listed in Table **6**. Yet a few special considerations deserve mention in this section.

Most problems due to contact lenses develop slowly and become manifest only after a variable interval. It is thus desirable to document the findings regularly with any of the numerous photographic and video systems now available for clinical use, with which the data may be digitally stored and statistically processed.

The improved safety of modern synthetic materials and lens care products has greatly lessened the risks associated with contact lenses, but wearers must nonetheless be followed up regularly for the prevention of ocular damage, and particularly of slow, cumulative damage over the long term.

Table **6**   Initial visit or annual follow-up examination of the contact lens patient
General medical history, ocular history
Lids
Conjunctiva
Cornea
Sclera
Anterior chamber
Pupillary mobility
Crystalline lens
Vitreous body
Fundus
Visual fields
Refractive correction (objective, subjective)
Visual acuity
Binocular vision
Corneal diameter
Corneal thickness
Corneal topography
Tear flow
Intraocular pressure (in all patients over age 40 and those with progressive myopia, suspected glaucoma, or a positive family history)

Ocular examination before, during, and after contact lens fitting thus serves not only for the immediate detection of acute complications, but also for the early detection of incipient long-term complications, which may affect either the anatomy or the physiology of the eye. We therefore recommend adherence to the classical sequence of the routine ophthalmological examination: visual acuity, motility, lids, conjunctiva, cornea, anterior and posterior chambers, retina, and intraocular pressure.

Not only the eyes, but also the contact lenses should be examined. Any abnormalities of lens position, surface depositions, staining, defects, and changes in parameters should be noted. Microbiological tests may reveal poor lens hygiene and an elevated risk of infection. One should also try to determine whether the patient has a proper understanding of lens care. Dirty hands or a dirty lens case indicate that this is not so.

Lid

Inadequate opening or closure of the eyelids, excessive blinking, or blepharospasm will be immediately visible to the examiner without special equipment. Ordinary daylight is best for examination of the lids. A check for symmetry readily reveals any monocular abnormality, such as ptosis.

The normal interpalpebral space is almond-shaped and of equal height on the two sides. The lids snugly overlie the globe and point directly upward (lower lid) and downward (upper lid). The nasal canthus makes a sharp corner, while the temporal canthus is rounded. The lacrimal puncta are fully immersed in the lacrimal menisci.

The skin of the eyelids is very thin and elastic, and care must be taken to avoid injuring it when spreading the lids apart to insert contact lenses, particularly in infants and toddlers. Children's lids are soft and smooth, those of elderly persons baggy and wrinkled.

Pathological changes of the lids are often the first sign of an adverse reaction to the lens itself, or to lens disinfectants or cleaners. The skin between the lashes should be examined carefully with a slit lamp under high magnification to detect early reddening and scaling. These findings mandate discontinuation of the contact lenses, as they are predictive of toxic keratopathy, which does not appear till much later. Particular vigilance is required in patients with a history of squamous blepharitis, which predisposes to such problems and is thus a relative contraindication to the wearing of contact lenses.

Conjunctiva

The conjunctiva, an elastic, highly vascularized tissue lying in an exposed position between the globe and the lids, responds to all forms of irritation from within or without by vasodilatation, which is visible as conjunctival hyperemia (injection). This most common abnormal finding associated with contact lens problems often provides the key to their detection and differential diagnosis. Its location, extent, and type depend on the cause of irritation of the anterior segment, which may be mechanical, toxic, or metabolic, and may arise from the lens itself or from lens care products. The tarsal conjunctiva may display massive (follicular) swelling of the papillae in what is known as cobblestone conjunctivitis or giant papillary conjunctivitis (GPC).

Zones of conjunctival necrosis are occasionally seen. Inspection of the conjunctiva of the upper and lower lids is thus mandatory not only before fitting, but also at every follow-up examination.

Pathological changes of the bulbar conjunctiva range from simple injection to complex isolated or diffuse changes.

The form and distribution of any perilimbal injection in the area covered by a soft lens are important clues to the differential diagnosis, as are superficial and deep conjunctival vasodilatation and neovascularization. A circular impression from the lens on the conjunctiva is an early sign of tight lens syndrome (TLS) and should be carefully inspected and documented, as should any microerosions or hemorrhages under the surface of the lens. Fluorescein or rose bengal staining is helpful.

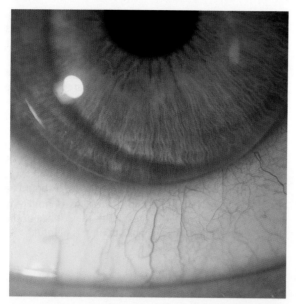

Fig. 1   Hard lens (PMMA), myopia, worn without problems for 20 years. Normal findings.

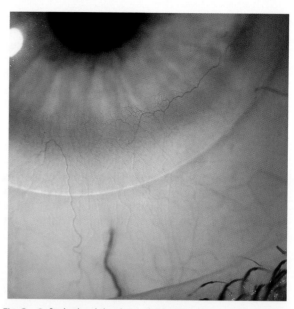

Fig. 2   Soft hydrophilic lens (hydroxymethyl methacrylate: HEMA), myopia, worn without problems for 10 years. Normal findings.

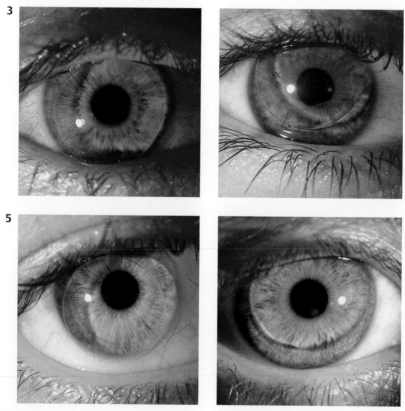

Fig. 3   Hard lens (fluorosilicone carbonate), high myopia, worn for 6 years without problems. Normal findings.

Fig. 4   Hard lens, hyperopia +7.5 diopter (D), worn without problems for 8 years. Normal findings.

Fig. 5   Absence of eye irritation, myopia, hard oxygen-permeable (RGP) CAB lenses worn for 8 years. Normal findings.

Fig. 6   Absence of eye irritation, keratoconus, spheric equivalent −16.25 D, CAB lens worn without problems for 13 years. Normal findings.

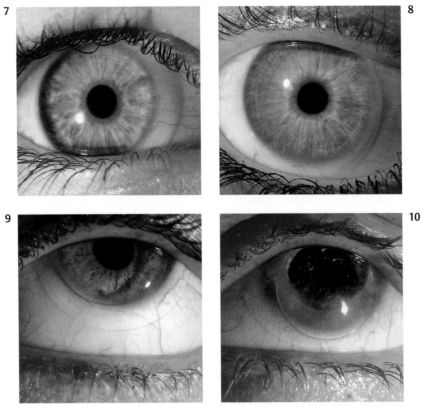

Fig. **7** Myopia, gel lens of high water content, worn without problems for 10 years. Normal findings.

Fig. **8** Myopia −3.75 D, disposable lenses worn without problems for 5 years. Normal findings.

Fig. **9** Absence of eye irritation, irregular astigmatism after photorefractive keratectomy (PRK). Piggyback system (hard lens on soft lens) worn for 3 years without complication.

Fig. **10** Aphakia, irregular astigmatism, previous iritis, complication cataract operation with secondary glaucoma. Piggyback system worn for 2 years without complication.

Cornea

The cornea is inspected in the usual manner, with a slit lamp, before and after removal of the contact lens. First, the position and mobility of the lens are examined under low magnification. Tear lenses are more easily examined after instillation of a fluorescein solution of suitable type. Fluorescein sodium, which is water-soluble, must not be used with soft gel lenses, as it will bind to them and cause permanent staining. High-molecular-weight fluorescein preparations are now available for use with gel lenses, but their fluorescence is much weaker than that of fluorescein sodium.

Rose bengal 2% is another useful dye for examination of the conjunctival and corneal epithelium after lens removal. Staining of epithelial cells may indicate a dry-eye condition associated with lens wearing. Rose bengal can bind to any type of synthetic material and thus is not routinely instilled when the contact lens is in place. Both fluorescein and rose bengal must be completely rinsed from the eye with sterile saline, and the lens should only be reinserted after a suitable interval, because even minute quantities of dye remaining in the conjunctival sac can stain it irreversibly.

The location and extent of neovascularization at the limbus indicate whether a metabolic, mechanical, or toxic disturbance is present. These vessels are best seen with slit-lamp illumination at 10–20 × magnification under red-free light.

Fine defects in the epithelium or stroma can be seen with a slit lamp at high magnification only; we recommend 30 ×. Examination of the endothelium requires either an additional noncontact optical device for magnification up to 200 ×, or an endothelial contact lens. The latter provides better optics but requires removal of the patient's contact lenses, followed by the application of local anesthetic and coupling gel. Because these substances can damage the patient's contact lenses, there should be an interval of at least 4 hours before reinsertion.

The corneal curvature and thickness should be measured regularly, as they may slowly change under the gentle pressure exerted by contact lenses, whether hard or soft. Irregular astigmatism, occurring after years or decades of wear, can make returning to spectacles very difficult and may also impede refractive corneal surgery. A rapid change of corneal curvature is the result, either of an orthokeratological effect, or of flat fitting. Changes of corneal thickness imply an adverse mechanical and physiological effect of contact lens wearing.

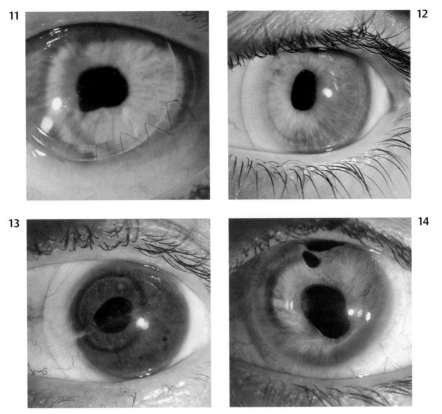

Fig. **11** Aphakia after bulbar perforation in a 4-year-old child. High (Dk) RGP lens +25 D, 3 months of problem-free wearing, corneal sutures in place. No sign of irritation.

Fig. **13** Traumatic aphakia and astigmatism after perforating injury (stabbing). Soft lens worn without complication for 13 years, no ocular irritation.

Fig. **12** Aphakia after early operation for congenital cataract, image obtained 3 months after surgery. Disposable lens of high water content, +38 D, absence of eye irritation.

Fig. **14** Absence of eye irritation, aphakia, soft lenses worn without complication for 22 years.

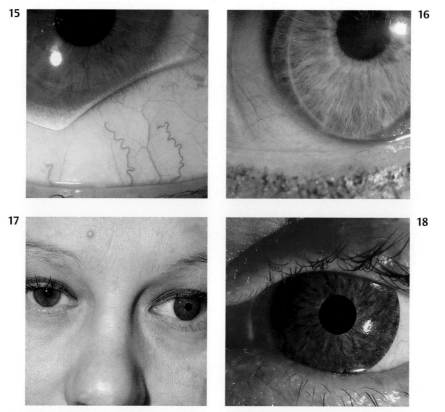

Fig. **15** Myopic astigmatism 7.0 D, truncated toric gel lens worn for 10 years without complication.

Fig. **16** High myopia and astigmatism, scleral PMMA lens −29 D worn for 38 years without complication, no eye irritation.

Fig. **17** Perforated bulb, traumatic aniridia, aphakia, and secondary glaucoma. Handpainted iris on gel lens worn for 9 years for cosmetic reasons.

Fig. **18** Same lens as in Figure **17**. Slightly dried surface, no other abnormalities, no problems with wear.

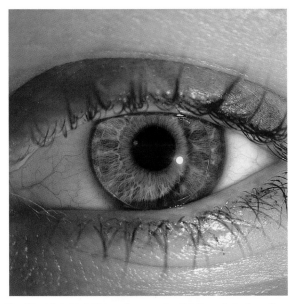

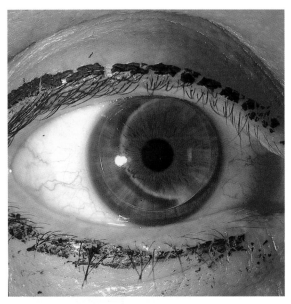

Fig. **19** High Dk RGP lens for myopia −3.0 D, no irritation after 20 hours of wearing.

Fig. **20** High Dk RGP lens for high myopia −17.0 D, no untoward findings after 19 hours of wear.

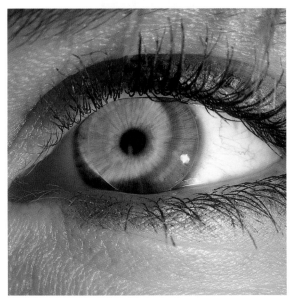

Fig. **21** RGP lens after 18 hours of wear, fitted for keratoconus, no irritation. Normal findings.

22

23

24

25

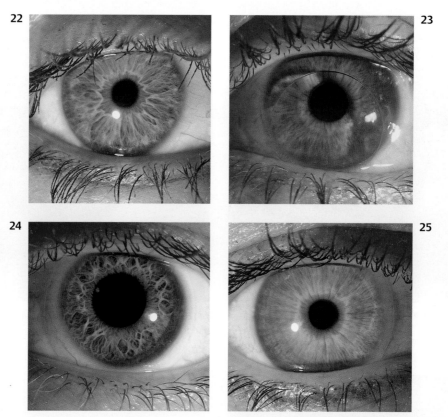

Fig. **22** Myopia −2.75 D, no irritation after 24 hours of uninterrupted wear.

Fig. **24** Soft lens for hyperopia +3.75 D after 28 hours of wear. No irritation.

Fig. **23** Myopia −4.5 D, high Dk RGP lens after 30 hours of wear during air travel. Normal findings.

Fig. **25** Soft lens designed for month-long wear. Worn for 24 hours without problems after 30 days of use. Normal findings.

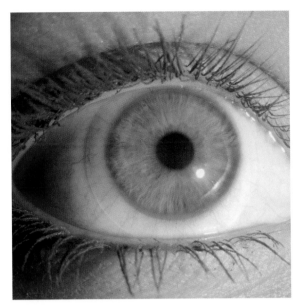

Fig. **26** Gel lens, high myopia –30.0 D, worn for 20 hours. Normal findings.

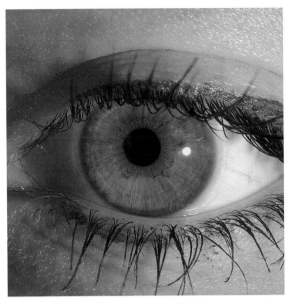

Fig. **27** Soft disposable lens after 30 days of use, no irritation after 42 hours of uninterrupted wear.

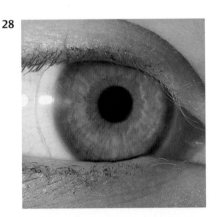

Fig. **28** Blue-green tinted plano lens worn for cosmetic reasons, no irritation after 24 hours of uninterrupted wear.

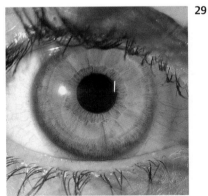

Fig. **29** Gel lens for myopia –3.25 D, tinted green for cosmetic reasons, no irritation after 10 hours of wear during a visit to a disco.

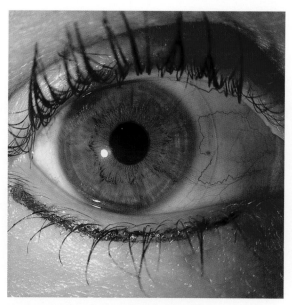

Fig. **30**   Extended-wear gel lens worn for medical reasons in the presence of chronically recurring corneal erosion. No untoward findings after 31 days of problem-free wear.

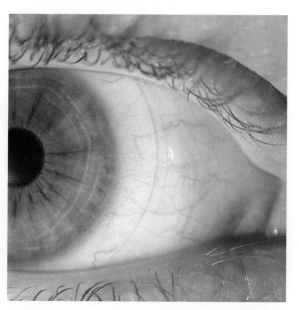

Fig. **31**   Soft hydrophilic lenses worn in piggyback mode (soft lens on another soft lens) to correct irregular astigmatism due to poor wound healing after an excimer laser operation. The patient was unable to wear hard lenses. The image, obtained after 21 days of wear, shows the absence of eye irritation.

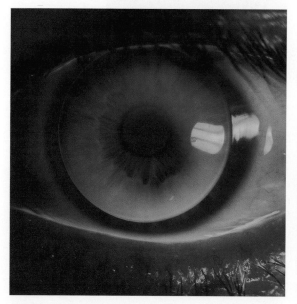

Fig. **32**   High Dk RGP lenses, myopia −12.5 D, fluorescein instilled for photography, lens well fitted, problem-free wear for 6 years.

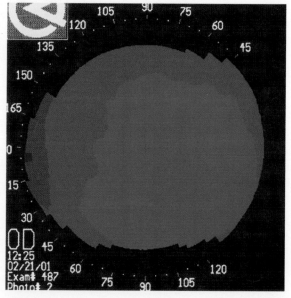

Fig. **33**   Same case as in Figure **32**. The corneal topographic image shows no deformation of the anterior surface and stable corneal radii for the entire duration of wear.

Inner Eye

The contact lenses must be removed for examination of the interior of the eye, because contact lens shadows, particularly from lenticular lenses, may create misleading appearances. Moreover, mydriatic drugs instilled to enable retinal examination can bind to certain types of contact lenses and, as they are slowly released, produce an undesired mydriasis, which may last for days.

Intraocular Pressure

The intraocular pressure (IOP) should be measured once or twice a year in all persons over 40, more often when there is a family history of glaucoma. The same applies to persons wearing contact lenses, particularly because raised IOP is a potential cause of corneal edema.

Any sudden change in refractive error in a patient wearing either spectacles or contact lenses, increased glare, or altered contrast suggests the possibility of raised IOP. As these are also the classic symptoms of damage due to contact lens wearing, a careful differential diagnostic evaluation is needed. If doubt persists, perimetry may help.

Just as in patients who do not wear contact lenses, the IOP is measured by applanation tonometry. The patient's contact lenses must be removed before the instillation of local anesthetic and fluorescein. To prevent binding of these potentially toxic and lens-damaging substances, the reinsertion of hard lenses should be delayed for at least 20 minutes, that of soft lenses for at least 2 hours.

Refractive Error and Visual Acuity

Refractive error and visual acuity (VA) should be measured both subjectively and objectively, just as in patients wearing spectacles, and any change should prompt a search for the cause (see p. 128).

The pressure exerted by a hard contact lens on the cornea can alter its topography (the so-called orthokeratologic effect). The corneal refractive power may be transiently altered and may not return to a stable value until weeks after the contact lens is removed. Measurement of the refractive error in the meantime may yield misleading results. Lenses fitted too steeply cause apparent worsening of myopia or improvement of hyperopia, while lenses fitted too flatly have the opposite effect.

If the patient wants a pair of spectacles for brief, occasional use but plans to continue wearing contact lenses at other times, a prescription for average spherical values will be a satisfactory compromise. In patients who must stop wearing contact lenses because of incipient presbyopia, impending military service, or other reasons, the refractive error should be measured no less than 21 days after the contact lenses are removed, or else the spectacle prescription may turn out to be inaccurate.

Any difficulty in finding the correct prescription should be dealt with by objective refraction, with and without contact lenses. Automatic refractometers cannot be used with certain types of lenses, for a variety of reasons. For example, the measuring beam may be of a wavelength that is reflected, rather than transmitted, by the lens material, so that the measured refractive error will be incorrect. A skiascope or manual refractometer will help in such cases.

Binocular Vision

Good binocular vision requires that the eyes be parallel in primary gaze and have unimpaired motility. A patient who has good binocular vision while wearing spectacles will not necessarily have it while wearing contact lenses, even if they are optimally fitted. Movement of the contact lens over the cornea during lid opening and closure may impair image fusion, and the different accommodative effort needed when contact lenses are worn may bring out a latent or barely compensated strabismus. When a problem with fusion arises in a patient wearing contact lenses, and particularly in a hyperopic patient, the contact lenses should be suspected as the cause, and an orthoptic examination should be performed. A Pola test may also be helpful.

Inspection of Contact Lenses

Not only the patient, but also the contact lenses should be examined, as defective contact lenses frequently cause intolerable eye irritation and other complications. They are best inspected with a binocular dissecting microscope or a slit lamp fitted with a contact lens holder. All lenses should be checked for surface deposits, stains, cracks, tears, defects, and wavy deformations at their edges.

Deposits on the lenses may be an early sign of ocular damage or systemic disease and should be carefully classified and documented. For the detection of defects, the slit lamp is not as good as a dark-field device developed by Zeiss for this purpose. Deviations of the geometric and optical parameters of the lens (diameter, thickness, curvature, refractive index) may be looked for under polarized light but are, in general, hard to detect without equipment that is too specialized for most practices.

The position and movement of the contact lens on the cornea should be observed during vertical and horizontal eye movements, as well as lid opening and closure. The tolerance values for such movements depend on the type of lens.

Inspection of Contact Lens Cases

The contact lens case should be regularly inspected and its condition recorded. Dirty, leaky, or stained cases can cause ocular infection.

Disinfectant solution may be less effective if there are air bubbles between the lens and lens case, if the well is incompletely filled, or if the fluid itself is discolored. Repeated topping-off of the disinfectant solution instead of emptying and refilling with fresh solution at each use may cause gradual accumulation of toxic substances, and, ultimately, toxic keratopathy.

Proper evaluation of a corneal ulcer requires obtaining a swab for bacterial culture not only of the eye, but also of the lens case. A positive culture from the lens case suggests poor compliance with the recommended lens care routine. Not only is such a finding important for patient care, it may also benefit the ophthalmologist should the corneal ulcer become the object of a lawsuit.

Documentation of Findings

Ocular findings are most easily documented on the special file cards provided by contact lens manufacturers. More modern methods of data storage on videotape, computer diskette, or CD-ROM have the advantage of enabling retrieval of earlier slit-lamp images for direct visual comparison with current findings. Sometimes, newly detected pathological conditions will turn out to have been overlooked on earlier examinations.

Patients can be registered by code number, and verbal descriptions can be stored along with the images. The video data can be digitized for electronic processing. In the future, the complete set of digitized images of each contact-lens wearer will be stored and evaluated by computer, and statistical analysis will yield information of both clinical and scientific interest. Even today, images are routinely transmitted over the Internet for assessment in centers with special expertise in the diagnosis and treatment of contact lens complications.

Follow-up

Every new fitting of contact lenses should be preceded by an ophthalmological examination, so that the potential complications of lens fitting and wearing can be avoided. In fact, studies of unsuccessful fitting have shown that the cause of failure could often have been identified beforehand.

Ophthalmologists agree that most serious complications can be prevented by examination of the patient before fitting to detect risk factors, and by more careful medical follow-up afterward. The preliminary and follow-up examinations must be conscientious and thorough, with attention not only to the eye, but also to the general medical history and review of systems.

The proper timing and frequency of follow-up depend on the type of lens and mode of wear. Patients who wear their lenses only occasionally, as during athletic activities, need the least frequent follow-up, while, for example, visually impaired babies whose lenses will be in place for days or weeks at a time must be seen much more often.

Newborns should be seen daily, and infants once every 1–4 weeks. The contact lenses should not just be checked but also cleaned in the laboratory, or exchanged, if necessary. Particularly in aphakic babies, the condition of the eye and the refractive index must be rechecked at short intervals, so that the geometric and optical parameters of the lenses can be properly adjusted.

Follow-up visits can be more widely spaced as the child grows older. Once the age of 12 months is reached, follow-up can be once every 4–6 weeks, and later once every 3 months. The same frequency of follow-up is needed for adult wearers of extended-wear lenses.

School-age children and adolescents should be seen every 3–6 months, depending on mode of wear; adults wearing hard or soft lenses should visit the ophthalmologist roughly twice a year, or once a year if they wear lenses only occasionally. Yearly examinations are needed in any case for glaucoma screening.

Patients at high risk of complications, such as those with diabetes, allergies, or AIDS or those undergoing chemotherapy, should be seen more frequently, as should adolescents whose prescription is rapidly changing. Patients with seasonal illnesses, such as hay fever or corneal herpes (which worsen during damp periods), should be seen more frequently in the corresponding seasons.

Table **7**   Interval between follow-up examinations

Age of patient	Contact lens type and mode of wear		
	Hard lenses	Soft lenses Daily wear	Extended wear
0–14 days	–	Daily	Daily
< 3 months	–	1 week	1 week
< 3 years	–	3 months	1 month
< 10 years	3 months	3 months	1 month
< 18 years	6 months	3 months	3 months
Adult	6–12 months	3–6 months	3 months

3 Pathologic Findings

Lid

Anatomy and Physiology

Increased Lid Tension and Blepharospasm

Ptosis

Lid Swelling and Edema

Infectious Blepharitis, Squamous Blepharitis, Ulceration

Lid injury

Conjunctiva

Anatomy and Physiology

Tarsal Conjunctiva

Bulbar Conjunctiva

Sclera

Anatomy and Physiology

Pathology

Cornea

Anatomy and Physiology

Epithelial Changes

Stromal Changes

Changes of Descemet's Membrane and the Endothelium

Topographic Changes

Inner Eye

Iritis, Uveitis, Panophthalmitis

Cataract

Intraocular Hypertension, Glaucoma

Retinal Diseases and Detachment

Lid

Anatomy and Physiology

The lids are composed of skin, cartilage, connective tissue, and muscle. The lid muscles not only enable blinking, but also, as a component of the mimetic musculature, communicate the emotional state of the individual. Normal lid function is very important in contactology. With each blink, the surface of the eye is covered with the salt-rich aqueous secretion of the lacrimal glands, and with the fatty secretion of the Meibomian glands that are found at the lid margins.

Normal blinking is involuntary and rhythmic when the eyes are adequately wetted, and more frequent when they are dry. Tear flow increases in response to irritation. Chronic excessive tear flow is due to partial or total obstruction of the lacrimal pathway or to an abnormal position of the lid.

The most important tasks of the lid are to prevent drying, visual glare, and ocular injury. These tasks depend upon normal lid function, especially in the contact lens wearer. Each blink distributes the tear fluid over the anterior surface of the contact lens and simultaneously slides the contact lens up and down over the cornea, thus enabling exchange of tear fluid in the space between the corneal surface and the posterior surface of the contact lens, the so-called tear lens. Lid closure also cleans the contact lens of any particulate foreign matter deposited on its surface through the tear fluid, or from the ambient environment.

The skin of the lid may suffer from any ailment known to dermatology. The most common in contact lens wearers is eczema, which tends to take the form of squamous blepharitis in patients suffering from allergic or ectopic dermatitis. Allergic reactions can be induced both by the lens itself and by the chemicals in lens care products.

Increased Lid Tension and Blepharospasm

Symptoms: Uncontrollable bilateral lid contraction.

Clinical findings: Lid opening, whether active or passive, is difficult or even impossible.

Every contact lens fitter is familiar with the reflex increase in lid pressure and spasmodic lid closure that are often encountered during the initial fitting phase. Failure to improve over time may make the further wearing of contact lenses impossible. These problems are less likely to occur with soft lenses.

Blepharospasm with excessive tearing, appearing after a period of unproblematic lens wear, should always be considered abnormal (see Table **8**). It is usually caused by acute mechanical irritation of the anterior segment, as by a crack or tear in the lens or by a lesion of the lid margin, conjunctiva, or cornea. Severe inflammation or infection, or a foreign body, can also cause increased lid pressure and blepharospasm.

Prophylaxis: Blepharospasm appearing soon after fitting in the sensitive patient can be reduced by having the patient wear the lenses for only a short time each day at first, and then for gradually longer times. Regular lens replacement lessens the frequency of lens defects and thus prevents the mechanical irritation that they cause.

Differential diagnosis: Aside from the factors already mentioned, blepharospasm may also be caused by neurological or psychiatric disease. Sometimes it is caused by glare, particularly in children undergoing slit-lamp examination.

> **Note:** There is no specific treatment for blepharospasm. If a contact lens is to be removed from a blepharospastic eye, it may be helpful to instill a local anesthetic first. (Caution: gel lenses will absorb the anesthetic agent and must, therefore, be discarded afterward.)

Table **8**   Causes of blepharospasm in contact lens wearers
Break-in period
Excessive lens mobility
Defective lens
Slipped or inverted lens
Irregularities or deposits on the lens surface
Dry eye, tear deficiency syndrome
Infection or injury of the lids, conjunctiva, or cornea
Foreign bodies of any type
Psychogenic

Ptosis

Symptoms: The upper lid cannot be adequately elevated.

Clinical findings: The upper lid overlaps the limbal area of the cornea regardless of the direction of gaze. Severe ptosis may impair vision.

Ptosis is usually easy to recognize because of the narrowing of the palpebral fissure, which is most often unilateral, though of variable extent. The diagnosis is made by observing that the midpoint of the upper lid is not contiguous with the upper edge of the pupil, but partially or completely overlaps the pupil when the patient looks straight ahead. If more than half of the pupil is covered, vision will be considerably impaired and treatment will be required, perhaps involving a surgical procedure.

Ptosis occasionally occurs as a complication after hard contact lenses are worn for many years. Levator function is impaired by chronic irritation due to the contact lens. This form of ptosis is thus often accompanied by decreased tearing, chronic conjunctivitis, or conjunctival scarring. Scarring is usually seen in the setting of advanced giant papillary conjunctivitis (GPC) and is easy to observe when the lids are ectropionized.

Occasionally, supposedly lost contact lenses, or fragments thereof, can burrow into the subtarsal lid tissue and cause a ptosis, appearing months later.

Differential diagnosis: Neurological disorders, particularly myasthenia gravis, should be included in the differential diagnosis. Pseudoptosis due to blepharospasm can be tested for by instillation of local anesthetic, which abolishes it.

Prophylaxis: Ptosis can be prevented by changing the lenses regularly, and by not wearing them during periods of seasonal allergy.

> **Note:** Any ptosis that is not due to contact lenses warrants neurological examination.

Lid Swelling and Edema

Symptoms: Swelling of upper and lower lids, discomfort, and fatigue.

Clinical findings: Swollen, thickened lids.

In contrast to inflammatory or traumatic lid swelling, primary allergic lid edema in contact lens wearers is not accompanied by hyperemia. The upper and lower lids are markedly swollen, and the skin of the lids is devoid of its normal wrinkles. Gentle pressure with a fingertip produces an indentation that lasts for several minutes.

Lid edema has both internal and external causes; in contact lens wearers, it is usually caused by allergy to the lens or to lens care products. Artificial tears may soothe the discomfort of lid edema but are often themselves responsible for it.

Differential diagnosis: Aside from allergy to the lens and lens care products, lid edema may be caused by cardiovascular disease, renal failure, generalized allergy, and other systemic illnesses, and usually calls for general medical evaluation and treatment. Hyperacute lid swelling (Quincke's edema) is due to generalized allergy or to poisoning.

Prophylaxis: Persons suffering from allergies should not wear contact lenses during critical seasons or in allergen-rich environments.

> **Note:** Lid swelling of uncertain cause requires general medical evaluation.

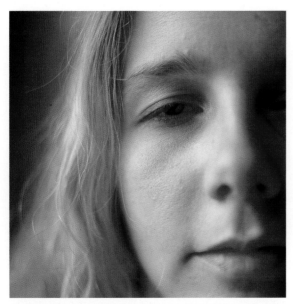

Fig. **34** Pseudoptosis due to chronic irritation after many years of wearing moderately well-tolerated hard lenses; an associated finding in a patient with GPC.

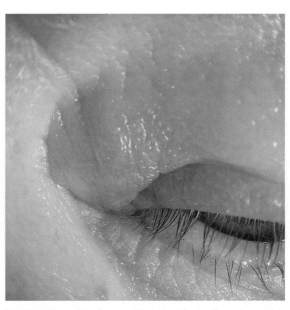

Fig. **35** Upper lid edema, soft contact lens, allergy to quaternary ammonium bases.

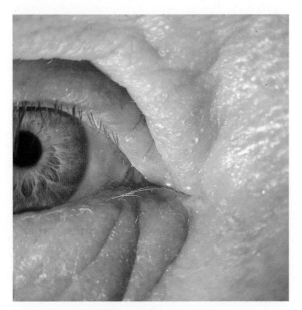

Fig. **36** Ectopic dermatitis of the lids; allergy to cobalt, nickel, synthetic materials, mercurial compounds and solutions.

Infectious Blepharitis, Squamous Blepharitis, Ulceration

Symptoms: Itching of the upper lid, especially the lid margins.

Clinical findings: Reddening and swelling of the lid skin; scaling, loss of lashes.

Infectious and allergic lid changes are usually seen in combination among contact lens wearers. Infectious blepharitis is usually secondary to a preceding allergic reaction. Squamous blepharitis is classically characterized by reddening, swelling, and scaling of the lid margins. Its causes and course are identical to that of localized eczema occurring elsewhere on the skin. Squamous blepharitis is sometimes restricted to the lid margins, in the spaces between the lashes. The lashes are brittle, poorly developed, or absent, and they may grow in an abnormal direction.

More severe blepharitis affects the entire surface of the lids and extends beyond them to the skin of the face. In severe cases, the skin in the region of the inner canthus is macerated or ulcerated. An allergy is always the cause; in contact lens wearers, the allergy may be to the contact lens, to lens care products, or to artificial tears. Blepharitis is particularly common in immunodeficient contact lens wearers (p. 160).

Superinfection is usually due to poor hygiene or an impaired immune response. The responsible organism is usually bacterial, though fungi are particularly common in immunocompromised persons, such as those with diabetes or AIDS. Almost all cases of superinfection are in wearers of soft contact lenses; hard lenses have a negligible absorptive capacity, and the material used to make them is better tolerated.

Differential diagnosis: Any other cause of dermatitis may be responsible, as may an allergy to any other substance in the environment, e.g., in cosmetics or environmental toxins. Other possibilities include dermatoses, irritation from a hordeolum or chalazion, basal cell carcinoma, and epithelioma.

Prophylaxis: Patients predisposed to blepharitis should not wear contact lenses. Preservative-free lens care products may help reduce its incidence.

> **Note:** Recurrent blepharitis requires evaluation by an allergist or dermatologist.

37

38

39

40

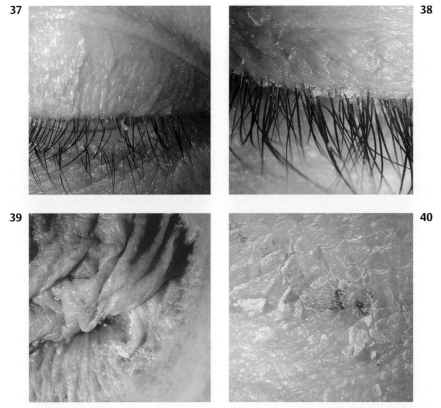

Fig. **37** Squamous blepharitis of unknown cause; mild form.

Fig. **38** Squamous blepharitis caused by chlorhexidine-containing lens care solution.

Fig. **39** Marked allergic blepharitis; wrinkling of the corner of the lid due to HEMA allergy.

Fig. **40** Eczema of the upper lid; allergy to PVP.

41

42

43

44

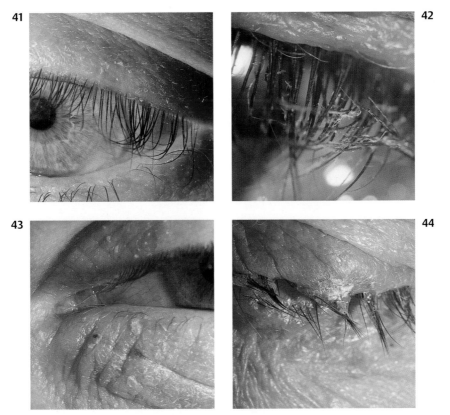

Fig. **41** Eczema of upper and lower lids; allergy to benzalkonium chloride (BAC) and chlorhexidine.

Fig. **43** Marked upper and lower lid eczema caused by allergy to chlorbutanol, thiomersal, and BAC.

Fig. **42** Matting of the upper lid cilia due to recurrent blepharitis.

Fig. **44** Blepharoconjunctivitis; purulent crusting on the lashes; typical problem caused by bad hygiene.

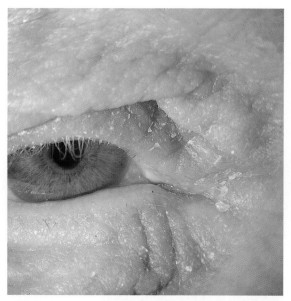

Fig. 45 Bacterial blepharoconjunctivitis with staphylococcal superinfection.

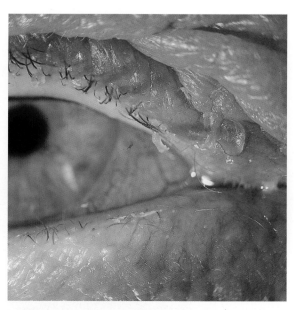

Fig. 46 Swelling of upper and lower lids; allergic blepharitis; allergy to thiomersal and BAC; bacterial superinfection.

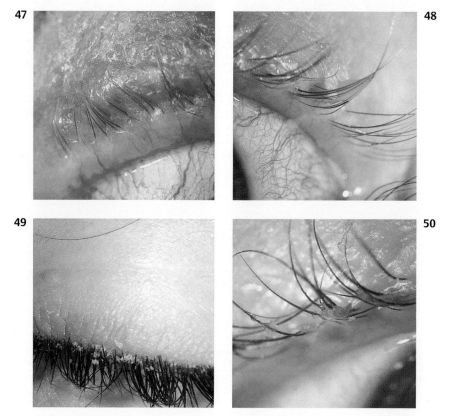

Fig. 47 Marked lower lid dermatitis in gel lens wearer with severe diabetes mellitus; epithelial scaling; superinfection with *Candida*.

Fig. 49 Ectopic dermatitis; scaling along the lid margin; allergy to cosmetics and contact lens products.

Fig. 48 Allergic blepharoconjunctivitis in an aphakic eye; superinfected with *Haemophilus*; intraocular inflammation.

Fig. 50 Bacterial blepharitis; conjunctivitis; purulent material seeping through the lashes on the upper lid.

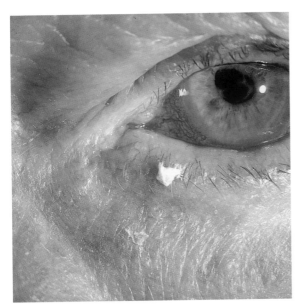

Fig. **51** Typical squamous blepharitis with scaly deposits on the lashes; allergy to penicillin and thiomersal.

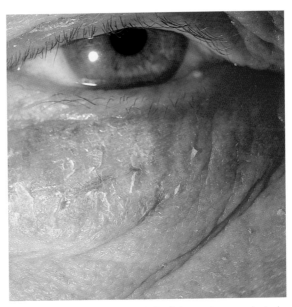

Fig. **52** Bacterial infection of the lid margins; purulent deposits on the lashes; staphylococcal infection in contact lens wearer with AIDS.

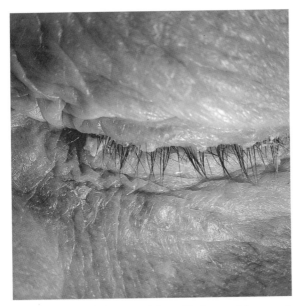

Fig. **53** Severe blepharitis with loss of lashes; nodular concretions of the lipid-secreting glands on the lid margin, caused by allergy to lens care products. Further testing revealed a nickel allergy (intolerance to piercing).

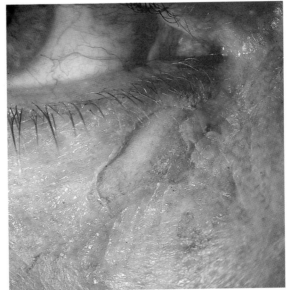

Fig. **54** Ulceration of the lower lid at the inner canthus; severe allergy to multiple preservative agents and lens materials, cobalt allergy, intolerance to piercing.

Lid Injury

Symptoms: Lid pain. When the lid margin is involved, there is a foreign-body sensation on opening or closing of the lids.

Clinical findings: Tissue defect, bleeding.

The inner surface of the lid and the tarsal conjunctiva are often injured by the edges of defective lenses. These injuries, though usually superficial, may nevertheless cause permanent scarring that impairs the function of the lid, leading to chronic corneal erosion or recurrent keratitis.

Defective soft corneoscleral lenses are particularly likely to injure the sclera or cornea, in addition to the lid. The problem usually arises because the lenses are worn for longer periods than recommended (whether they are of the disposable or brief-wear variety, or are part of a system of exchangeable lenses).

The wearing of hard PMMA lenses for many years can also chronically traumatize the tarsal conjunctiva, leaving scars that may make further lens wearing intolerably uncomfortable.

Differential diagnosis: Injuries of the types discussed here may be due to foreign bodies other than contact lenses, or to accidents (see p. 186). An adequate history usually reveals the cause.

Prophylaxis: Patients should not wear their contact lenses for longer than recommended, and should check them for defects before each insertion. Defective contact lenses do not belong in the eye.

> **Note:** Any lid injury should prompt examination for a concomitant injury of the bulb.

Conjunctiva

Anatomy and Physiology

The conjunctiva reacts promptly to endogenous and exogenous irritants and is thus a sensitive indicator of contact lens complications. Practically any problem caused directly or indirectly by contact lenses is associated with conjunctival changes (though not all conjunctival changes are due to contact lenses). Lid disease caused by contact lenses is associated with changes of the tarsal conjunctiva, and corneal disease caused by contact lenses is associated with changes of the bulbar conjunctiva.

Changes of the lids and cornea should be sought whenever a contact lens wearer presents with conjunctivitis, because, in contact lens wearers, the lids, cornea, and conjunctiva constitute a functional unit. The complications that arise are generally due to a disturbance of the physiological, metabolic, and toxicological interrelationship of these three structures. This interrelationship is the central theme of contactological research and accounts for a major part of the ophthalmologist's work in caring for the contact lens-wearing patient.

The conjunctiva is a mucous membrane that extends from the lid margins to the limbal region of the globe. It is a well vascularized, translucent membrane with two portions, tarsal (palpebral) and bulbar. The tarsal conjunctiva is tightly bound to the underlying tissue on the inner surface of the lid, while the bulbar conjunctiva is more loosely applied to the sclera, except in the limbal area. The fornix (zone of transition between the tarsal and bulbar conjunctiva) lies at the most remote area of the surface of the eyeball and forms the base of the conjunctival sac (cul-de-sac).

The conjunctiva is a mucous membrane containing many secretory cells; the most important of these for contact lens wearers are the goblet cells. When their function is impaired, lacrimation becomes deficient, the eye dries out, and a foreign body sensation ensues that makes lens-wearing intolerable.

Tarsal Conjunctiva

Follicular Swelling, Papillary Hypertrophy, Giant Papillary Conjunctivitis

Symptoms: Severe itching while wearing lenses; burning; increased secretions; impaired visual acuity (VA).

Clinical findings: Hyperemia, follicular swelling; papillary hypertrophy of the tarsal conjunctiva; recurrent deposition of hydrophobic material on lens surfaces.

Hyperemia, follicular swelling, and papillary hypertrophy of the tarsal conjunctiva are the classic signs of GPC in contact lens wearers, a complication that is not at all rare in wearers of hard or soft lenses. This condition is becoming significantly more common, not least because of air pollution.

Both in etiology and in phenotype, GPC resembles vernal conjunctivitis (vernal catarrh), a condition seen in the springtime in patients with an allergic predisposition. GPC is caused by proteins from the lacrimal fluid that are presumably denatured by lens-hygiene solutions and thereby become immunologically active. Deposited on the surface of the lens, these proteins act as antigens, to which antibodies then bind. The sandwich of lens, antigen, and antibody rubs on the tarsal conjunctiva, causing increased conjunctival swelling and secretions—the vicious cycle of GPC.

The hallmark of GPC is the coating of the contact lens surface with a strongly adherent protein layer, which pierces the film of tear fluid over the lens within seconds of insertion, leading to diminished visual acuity and increased glare. The case history generally points to the diagnosis: The patient wears lenses without complications for weeks or months and then, suddenly, a problem develops. A few minutes after lens insertion the patient experiences burning, chafing, and itching in the eyes. Tears and a film deposited on the surface of the lens impair visual acuity within a few seconds after the eyes are opened, and until the next blink. Conjunctival secretions cause the eyelids to stick together and limit the mobility of the contact lens during blinking and eye movements.

Examination reveals the following: the contact lens is barely mobile or immobile on the surface of the eye and is coated with a grayish-white film that makes it look dry and dull. The lids are mildly swollen, and their margins are coated with dried yellowish-white secretion. The bulbar conjunctiva is mildly injected; everting the lids reveals a massive papillary swelling of the tarsal conjunctiva, which is made even more evident with fluorescein staining. GPC can be classified into four stages (Table **9**).

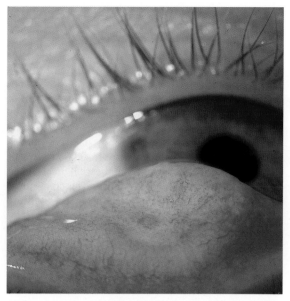 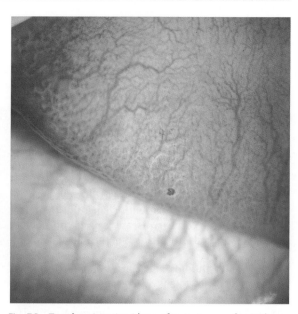

Fig. **55**   Scarring of the tarsal conjunctiva of the lower lid after decades of wearing hard PMMA lenses.

Fig. **56**   Tarsal conjunctiva 1 hour after test wear of a rigid contact lens for myopia; injection of conjunctival vessels.

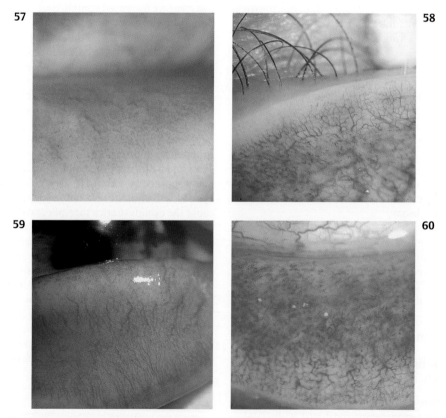

Fig. **57**   Isolated hyperemia of the upper lid conjunctiva caused by protein deposits on the anterior surface of a soft contact lens.

Fig. **59**   Injection of the upper lid conjunctiva; focal conjunctival atrophy after 18 years of wearing hard lenses for keratoconus; tear deficiency.

Fig. **58**   Mild hyperemia of the tarsal conjunctiva; mechanical irritation of the conjunctiva on the initial fitting of a hard lens.

Fig. **60**   Upper-lid hyperemia and edema; allergic reaction to chlorhexidine.

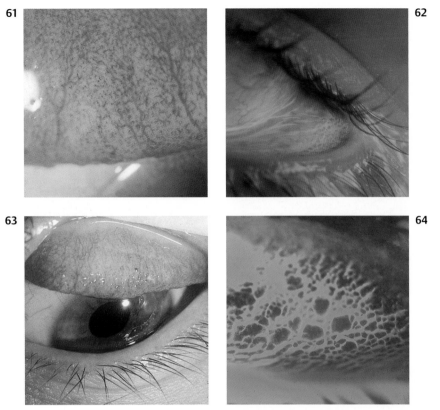

Fig. **61**   Upper-lid hyperemia; mild cockscomb swelling of the conjunctiva indicating chronic irritation; hard contact lens worn for 6 years.

Fig. **63**   GPC reaction on upper lid; marked hypertrophy of the papillae; hyperemia.

Fig. **62**   Early GPC, characterized by hyperemia and moderate papillary hypertrophy; soft hydrophilic lens.

Fig. **64**   GPC stage 1–2; isolated tarsal conjunctival hyperemia; papillary hypertrophy in the region of the fold.

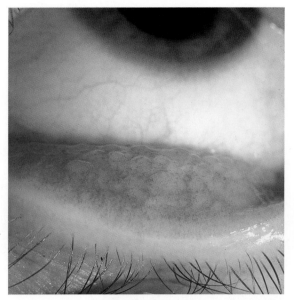

Fig. **65**   GPC stage 2–3; papillary hypertrophy; identical picture to vernal conjunctivitis.

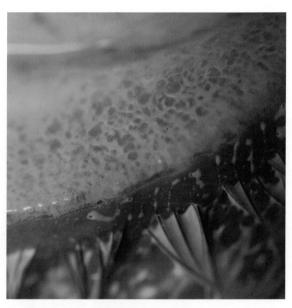

Fig. **66**   GPC in a CAB lens wearer; stage 2; fluorescein staining.

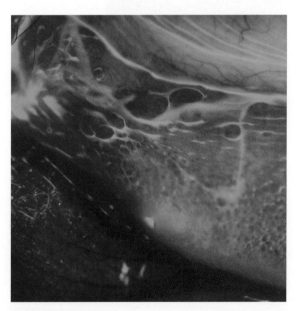

Fig. **67**   GPC follicular swelling in the region of the lower conjunctival fold; soft contact lens worn for 3 months.

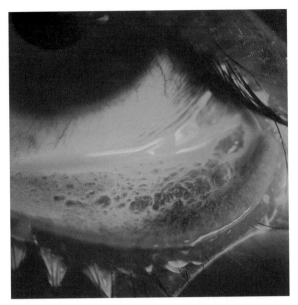

Fig. **68** GPC stage 3; fluorescein staining; PMMA lens worn for 11 years.

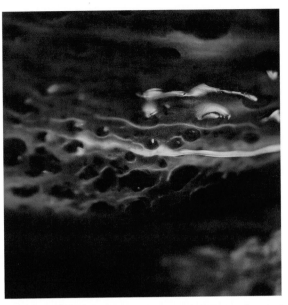

Fig. **69** Marked GPC, stage 3; fluorescein staining; gel contact lens worn for 4 months.

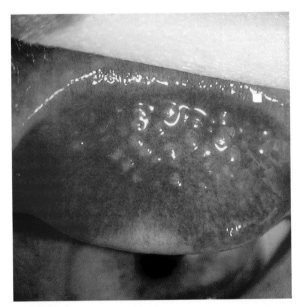

Fig. **70** GPC; scarring; 9 months of wearing a fluorosilicone carbonate lens.

Table **9**   Stages of giant papillary conjunctivitis

Stage	Papillary appear-ance	Mucus	Lens wearing comfort	Visual acuity with lens
1	Little change	Minimal	Good	Very good
2	Diameter up to 0.5 mm	Moderate	Slightly decreased	Still good
3	Diameter up to 0.7 mm	Moderate	Markedly decreased	Variable
4	Diameter greater than 0.7 mm	Copious	Lenses un-wearable	Markedly diminished

Differential diagnosis: Other conditions resembling GPC include other allergic reactions of the conjunctiva, auto-immune conditions, and (typically in the springtime) primary vernal conjunctivitis independent of the wearing of contact lenses.

Prevention: Meticulous daily lens hygiene, frequent use of protein removers, and a temporary cessation of lens wearing during critical seasons will reduce the risk of GPC.

Note: Patients with pollen allergy should be instructed not to wear contact lenses during the hay fever season.

Bulbar Conjunctiva

Conjunctival Edema and Acute Chemosis

Symptoms: Severe itching and tearing; difficulty closing the lids.

Clinical findings: Marked swelling of the conjunctiva that may project beyond the lid margin, with clear or san-guineous secretion. Mild proptosis.

Conjunctival edema in contact lens wearers is usually due to lens-cleaning solutions, or to wetting solutions or artificial tears that are supposed to enhance wearing comfort. Acute conjunctival edema may occur as early as the fitting phase, particularly when relevant details of the case history are not obtained or disregarded, such as a previous episode of allergic blepharitis or conjunctivitis requiring treatment. Patients with certain types of allergies, for example to thiomersal, a common constituent of eye drops and contact lens solutions, also tend to develop acute conjunctival reactions when contact lenses are fitted.

Acute chemosis is a complication that usually appears within a few minutes of the initial insertion of a lens or the initial use of a lens care product or variety of eye drops. Most of the affected patients were previously treated at some time with eye drops or ointments and were presumably sensitized in this way. An adequate history helps to identify and prevent this problem: patients should be asked at the initial prefitting visit whether they have ever had complications from the use of eye drops or ointments, or difficulty tolerating them. If so, the risk is high that the initial insertion of contact lenses will cause marked conjunctival swelling within minutes, so that the fitting will have to be terminated.

One can also use the Ophthalmotest to predict adverse reactions in advance and determine the offending solution constituent (cf. p. 80, 86).

Ophthalmologists periodically see an emergency case of acute chemosis referred by a contact-lens-fitting optician. The problem typically arises during a fitting session, for example on initial application of a wetting solution to improve lens-wearing comfort. Within a few minutes, massive conjunctival swelling in both eyes may completely occlude the palpebral fissure and make it difficult to close the lids. A retrospectively obtained history usually reveals that the patient has been using non-prescription eye drops irregularly over the years, without medical supervision, to treat hay fever or other allergic symptoms. Acute chemosis can occur even if eyedrops were last used years earlier.

Slit-lamp examination in acute chemosis reveals slightly thickened lids with mildly erythematous margins. The bulbar conjunctiva is severely swollen, and there is a large volume of clear or sanguineous secretion. The swelling extends beyond the lid margins, hindering lid closure. Corneal changes are only mild: there may be mild edema, and slit-lamp examination after fluorescein instillation may reveal fine stippling of the epithelium. The anterior chamber is usually normal, and, unless hindered by the swollen lids, vision is normal but for a slight increase in glare.

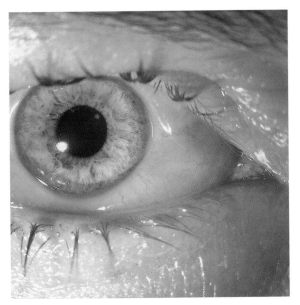

Fig. **71** Acute chemosis 45 seconds after insertion of a soft contact lens stored in Polyquad; known allergy to quaternary ammonium bases.

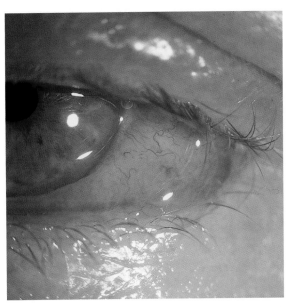

Fig. **72** Acute hemorrhagic chemosis after the application of an artificial tear solution to a dry eye; hard lens; BAC allergy.

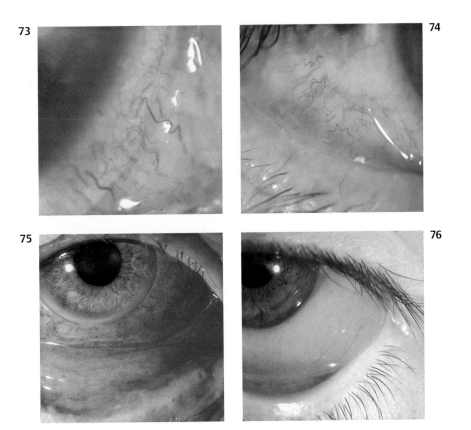

Fig. **73** Acute bulbar conjunctival injection; immediate reaction to PMMA lens; because of the pressure exerted by the contact lens, the edema is limited to the area *not* covered by the lens.

Fig. **75** Jelly-like swelling of the tarsal and bulbar conjunctiva after many years of astringent eye drop abuse while wearing soft contact lenses.

Fig. **74** Acute bulbar conjunctival injection; immediate reaction to chlorhexidine and thiomersal; the lens contact zone remains visible for a few minutes after the lens is removed.

Fig. **76** Acute chemosis in a gel lens wearer with known allergies to various plant species, after a brief stay in a garden. Remnants of organic foreign matter in the cul-de-sac, pollen dust on the lens surface.

Differential diagnosis: Acute chemosis can also occur as an allergic reaction to pollen, environmental pollutants, or other substances. Other causes include retrobulbar masses, severe intraocular infections, and radiation injury to the eyes.

Prophylaxis: Acute chemosis can often be prevented by meticulous history-taking.

> **Note:** When acute chemosis occurs, its cause must be determined before the lenses are worn again or new lenses are fitted; otherwise, a recurrence is likely.

Subconjunctival Hemorrhage

Symptoms: Usually no pain or discomfort, but patients are highly distressed by the prominently visible abnormality.

Clinical findings: Deep-red hematoma under the conjunctiva, which is usually somewhat raised.

Multiple microhemorrhagic spots are often present in the conjunctiva of contact lens wearers, usually in the perilimbal region where the lens rests, but occasionally in the tarsal conjunctiva. These easily visible lesions appear spontaneously, often sending the highly distressed patient to the emergency service of the eye clinic. There is usually no pain or impairment of visual acuity.

Blood begins to pool under the bulbar conjunctiva shortly after lens insertion, usually arising from a site of injury near the limbus and spreading out evenly under the conjunctiva of the lower half of the eye. When a soft lens is still on the eye, the hematoma in the area covered by the lens is somewhat compressed and thus paler than elsewhere. There is no pain, discomfort, or corneal edema, unless the eyes are rubbed.

High-power slit-lamp examination reveals the source of the bleeding as a small tear of the bulbar conjunctiva, rarely more than 1 mm long. Such tears often result from improper lens insertion or removal. Other causes are long fingernails or devices used for lens insertion or removal. Another common cause is a defect of the rim of the lens, for example, a sharp-edged lens tear, breakage, or deposit. Such lesions are usually caused by hard lenses but can also be caused by inadequately rehy-

drated soft lenses, or by disposable lenses that are worn far beyond the recommended period, until they physically deteriorate. Excessively long wear of disposable lenses regularly produces breaks and tears in the lens, which can injure the lids, conjunctiva, and cornea; similar defects can be produced by improper handling, inadequate hygiene, or storage under excessively dry conditions. The most common causes of subconjunctival hemorrhage are listed in Table **10**.

To minimize the risk of subconjunctival hemorrhage, the contact lenses should be inspected under a dissecting microscope, or a slit lamp fitted with a contact-lens-holding device, at every follow-up visit.

Differential diagnosis: Subconjunctival hemorrhage has a unique appearance and is hardly likely to be confused with any other disorder. It may, however, appear for reasons unrelated to the wearing of contact lenses.

Prophylaxis: Patients should be instructed to discard any lenses with visible defects, and to take care not to cut the eye when inserting and removing the lens. Persons with hemorrhagic disorders of any kind should not wear contact lenses.

> **Note:** Whenever conjunctival hemorrhage occurs, the contact lenses should be inspected for defects. Patients with recurrent hemorrhages should undergo medical evaluation for a bleeding disorder.

Table **10** Causes of conjunctival hemorrhage in contact lens wearers

A Related to contact lenses
Material defects, inadequate polishing, edge defects
Improper lens insertion or removal
Surface deposits
B Not related to contact lenses
Mechanical irritation, strong eye-rubbing
Vascular sclerosis
Coagulopathy, leukemia
Iatrogenic (anticoagulation)
Tear deficiency syndrome

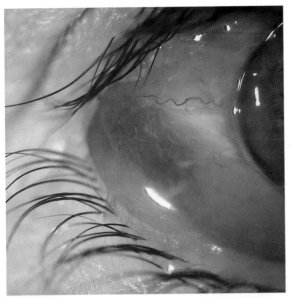

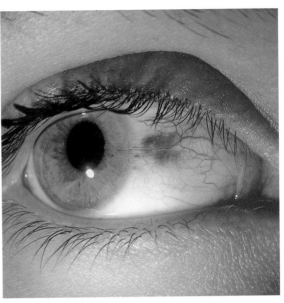

Fig. **77** Hyperacute, severe conjunctival edema; hemorrhagic form; immediate reaction after the initial insertion of a hard contact lens wetted with an artificial tear solution; longstanding abuse of astringent eye drops, known thiomersal allergy.

Fig. **78** Perilimbal hemorrhage of the bulbar conjunctiva caused by wearing a soft lens with edge defects.

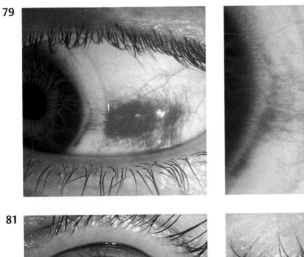

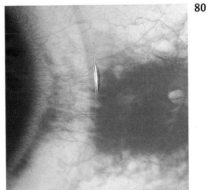

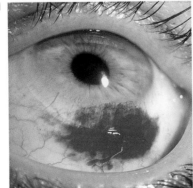

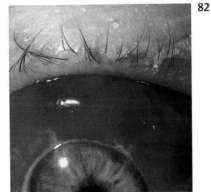

Fig. **79** Conjunctival lesion caused by wearing a disposable soft lens with an edge defect for several months longer than the recommended time.

Fig. **81** Extensive bleeding into the conjunctiva at the 6 o'clock position caused by an edge defect of a gel contact lens.

Fig. **80** Figure **79**, enlarged; the haptic of the gel lens acts as a tamponade for the hyposphagma.

Fig. **82** Massive conjunctival bleeding after wearing a hard contact lens with edge defects; 42-year-old patient with coagulopathy. Further wearing of contact lenses is contraindicated.

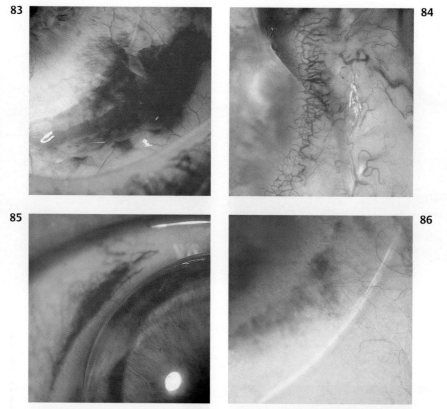

Fig. **83**   Cutting injury of the bulbar conjunctiva from a defective lens edge; disposable gel contact lens; prescribed wearing time exceeded.

Fig. **85**   Perilimbal, superficial conjunctival bleeding caused by improperly processed edge of a PMMA lens.

Fig. **84**   Cutting injury of the conjunctiva and cornea; 8-year-old soft hydrophilic corneoscleral lens *in situ;* large, sharp-edged defect.

Fig. **86**   Conjunctival hemorrhage in the sulcus region; mechanical irritation due to poor fitting.

Generalized Conjunctival Hyperemia

Conjunctival hyperemia in contact lens wearers has a variety of causes, which can often be distinguished from one another by the location and appearance of hyperemia. *Focal* conjunctival hyperemia is most often due to mechanical irritation of the conjunctiva in a circumscribed area from a dried-out, ill-fitted, defective, or deposit-coated lens; annular perilimbal injection is usually of toxic or allergic etiology. *Generalized* conjunctival hyperemia (i.e., of the entire conjunctiva, including the area under the contact lens) is usually caused by mechanical irritation or infection; other causes include inadequate lacrimation, allergic or toxic processes, and radiation injury. Whether focal or generalized, the hyperemic area is superficially discolored (brick-red); the reactively dilated vessels of the conjunctiva are always bright red and freely mobile over the scleral surface. (This is not so in cases of conjunctival hyperemia secondary to underlying deep or scleral infection.)

Mechanical Irritation and Injury

Symptoms: Eye-rubbing; foreign body sensation; tearing.

Clinical findings: The entire bulbar conjunctiva is injected and appears brick-red.

Conjunctival vasodilatation as a rapidly occurring response to a foreign body is routinely observed when a patient first starts to wear contact lenses. Surface vessels of the bulbar conjunctiva are greatly enlarged during this period. This response is normal in the initial phase of contact lens wear, but pathological at later times.

The causes of mechanical irritation of the conjunctiva in contact lens wearers are listed in Table **11**.

If a lens is fitted too flatly, its edge does not lie securely on the limbus and can rub against the conjunctiva. Lens cracks, fractures, or polishing defects, as well as surface deposits due to inadequate cleaning are other causes of mechanical irritation. Injury of the conjunctiva from an exogenous foreign body looks much the same as injury from a contact lens; the two situations may be difficult to distinguish. It may be useful to remove the lens and examine the conjunctiva with fluorescein or rose bengal staining; distinctive traces of the foreign body may become evident.

Table **11** Causes of mechanical irritation in contact lens wearers

Material defects, inadequate polishing
Flat fitting, decentration
Surface deposits
Lesion of the lid margin
Lesion of the cornea
Tear deficiency syndrome

A common cause of generalized conjunctival hyperemia in contact lens wearers is inadequate lacrimation. Any qualitative or quantitative, primary or secondary impairment of lacrimation impairs the ability of the lens to glide without friction over the cornea and conjunctiva. The unlubricated lens acts as a foreign body and causes mechanical conjunctivitis. The symptoms include burning, foreign body sensation, rubbing of the eye, and epiphora. Defects in the conjunctival and corneal epithelium can be detected with rose bengal.

Infection

Symptoms: Burning; eye-rubbing; foreign body sensation; epiphora.

Clinical findings: Injection and chemosis of the entire conjunctiva; secretions.

Conjunctivitis with generalized injection is certainly the most common complication of contact lens wearing. The symptoms include burning, foreign body sensation, eye-rubbing, and epiphora.

1. Bacterial Conjunctivitis

Symptoms: Burning; eye-rubbing; foreign body sensation; tearing.

Clinical findings: Generalized injection and chemosis; secretions in the cul-de-sac.

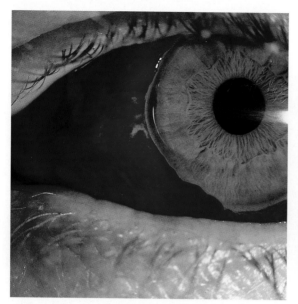

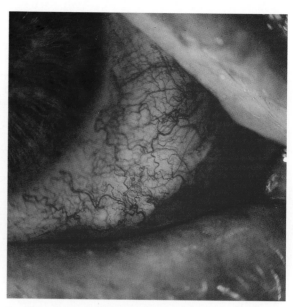

Fig. **87**   Severe conjunctival hemorrhage after a punch in the eye; the gel lens remained intact.

Fig. **88**   Conjunctival hyperemia; mechanical irritation from a hard contact lens characterized by an even, brick-red discoloration of the entire bulbar conjunctiva.

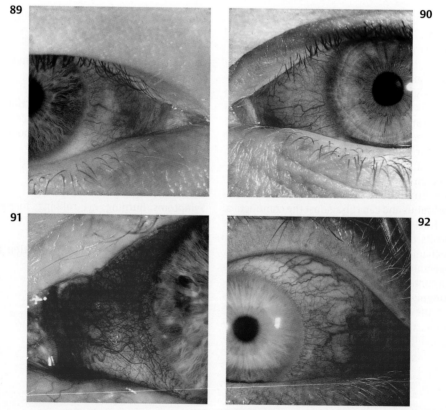

Fig. **89**   Focal lateral bulbar conjunctival hyperemia from a foreign body reaction; hard contact lens; typical brick-red color.

Fig. **91**   Focal limbal conjunctival hyperemia from a foreign body reaction; gel contact lens.

Fig. **90**   Focal lateral conjunctival hyperemia from a foreign body reaction; rigid contact lens.

Fig. **92**   Focal conjunctival hyperemia with accentuation near the limbus, due to a foreign body reaction; soft contact lens.

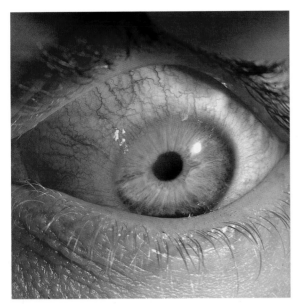

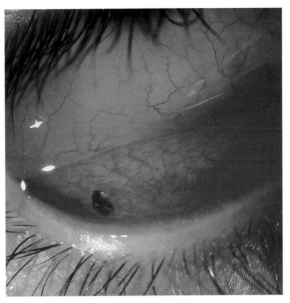

Fig. **93**   Diffuse conjunctival injection from a foreign body reaction to a rigid contact lens; tear deficiency.

Fig. **94**   Severe conjunctival swelling; erythema from a foreign body reaction in a patient wearing gel contact lenses. Eversion of the lower lid reveals an insect wing as the cause.

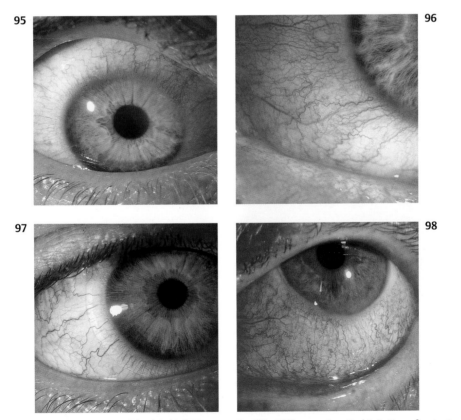

Fig. **95**   Diffuse conjunctival injection as a foreign body reaction to a hard contact lens worn for many hours.

Fig. **97**   Mild, diffuse conjunctival hyperemia; tear deficiency; gel contact lens with desiccated anterior surface.

Fig. **96**   Diffuse conjunctival irritation after test wear of a gel contact lens for 4 hours; tear deficiency.

Fig. **98**   Marked, deep-red conjunctival discoloration due to both superficial and deep vasodilatation; mechanical irritation; soft, hydrophilic contact lenses.

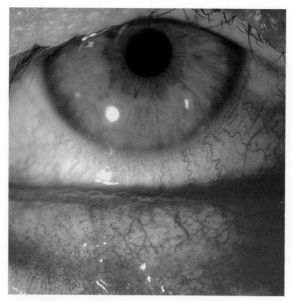

Fig. **99**   Marked, diffuse brick-red coloration of the conjunctiva in bacterial conjunctivitis.

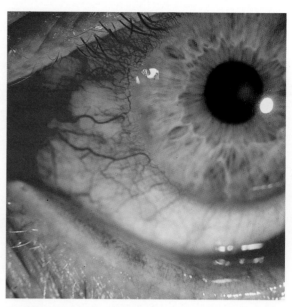

Fig. **100**   Bacterial conjunctivitis due to *Haemophilus* in a patient wearing gel contact lenses.

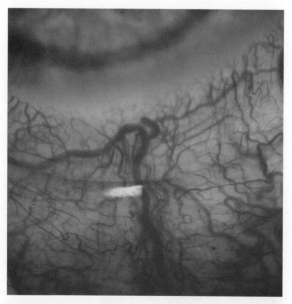

Fig. **101**   Massive conjunctival injection, mildly accentuated in the area contacted by the (soft, hydrophilic) contact lens; bacterial conjunctivitis due to *Pseudomonas*.

Table **12** Causes of conjunctivitis in contact lens wearers
Altered ocular flora
Epithelial defects
Faulty lens cleaning
Faulty lens disinfection
Tear deficiency
Elevated temperature of the corneal surface
Impaired immune competence
Chronic hypoxia
Overwearing
Wearing deteriorated lenses
Systemic infection
Wearing lenses during sleep
Parasitic infection

Table **13** The organisms that most frequently cause conjunctivitis in contact lens wearers

Adenovirus	Herpes simplex virus	Pneumococcus
Aspergillus	Haemophilus	Pseudomonas
Candida	Klebsiella	Staphylococcus
Chlamydia	Moraxella	

Infectious conjunctivitis is among the more common conditions treated by the ophthalmologist, affecting both contact lens wearers and the general population. Improper lens wear (Table **12**) predisposes to its occurrence; it is caused by a broad spectrum of microorganisms—bacteria, viruses, and occasionally fungi or *Acanthamoeba*.

The characteristic signs of bacterial conjunctivitis are swelling of the lids and generalized injection of the bulbar and tarsal conjunctivae. The cul-de-sac contains copious mucous or proteinaceous secretions. As long as the infection is limited to the conjunctiva, the cornea is clear and visual acuity is unaffected; the anterior chamber is normal. Excessive tearing may affect vision. If the interior of the eye is inflamed, changes in the refractive media may impair visual acuity, but this is rare. Culture of the secretions in the cul-de-sac may reveal the etiologic organism; *Pseudomonas, Staphylococcus, Haemophilus,* and *Pneumococcus* commonly cause conjunctivitis in contact lens wearers (Table **13**).

Bacterial conjunctivitis is often the result of inadequate lens hygiene. The biofilm in the lens case provides an excellent breeding ground for bacteria and fungi; soft, hydrophilic lenses are more commonly the vector of infection than hard lenses because their aqueous portion can act as a culture medium for microorganisms.

In patients with infectious conjunctivitis, samples for culture should be obtained not only from the cul-de-sac, but also from the surfaces of the contact lenses, and from the lens case, for identification of the organism and determination of its pattern of antibiotic sensitivity and resistance. The latter is particularly important, not only for the choice of the best antibiotic, but also for assessment of the efficacy of the various contact lens hygiene systems currently available on the market.

Differential diagnosis: Bacterial conjunctivitis is a clinically distinctive entity. It should not be forgotten, however, that conjunctivitis can be caused by foreign bodies of various kinds in the cul-de-sac, including "lost" contact lenses or lens fragments. Recurrent conjunctivitis may be due to an immunodeficient state, a metabolic disorder, or repeated reinfection from the throat, nose, skin, or ear (transfer of organisms by way of the pillow).

Prophylaxis: Two basic steps will minimize the risk of conjunctival inflammation: first do careful lens hygiene, second stop all lens wearing during an infection.

Note: Bacterial conjunctivitis in contact lens wearers is almost always due to poor lens hygiene. If lens-wearing is not discontinued, corneal infection may ensue.

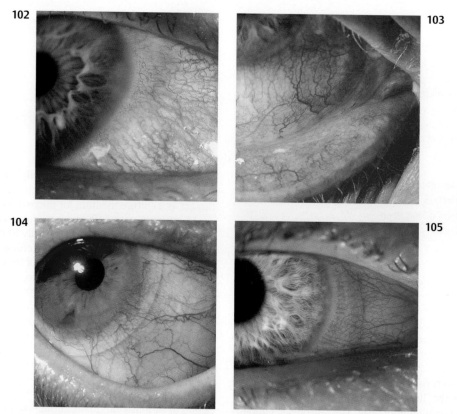

Fig. **102** Bacterial conjunctivitis; gel contact lens; diffuse conjunctival hyperemia without accentuation in the area contacted by the lens.

Fig. **104** Toxic hyperemia, most severe in the perilimbal area; thiomersal reaction; standard aphakic fitting.

Fig. **103** Bacterial conjunctivitis; soft contact lens; streptococcal infection.

Fig. **105** Mechanical hyperemia; perilimbal white ring of compression from steeply fitted lens; tear deficiency.

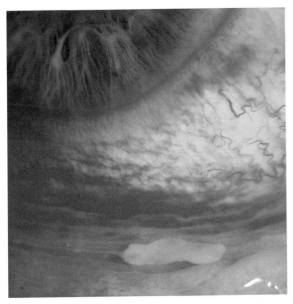

Fig. **106** Bacterial conjunctivitis; pus in the lower cul-de-sac; staphylococcal infection.

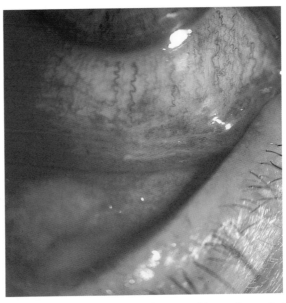

Fig. **107** Diffuse conjunctival infection and hemorrhage; viral conjunctivitis; hard contact lens.

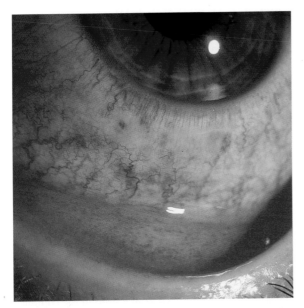

Fig. **108** Viral conjunctivitis; diffuse brick-red to deep-red discoloration of the conjunctiva, with hemorrhage; soft contact lens wearer.

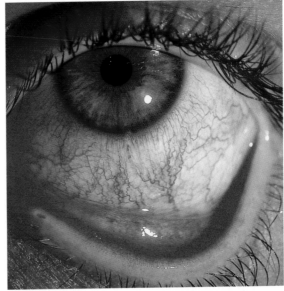

Fig. **109** Fungal conjunctivitis; diffuse vasodilatation with mild paralimbal accentuation; soft contact lens; candidiasis in a diabetic patient.

2. Viral Conjunctivitis

Symptoms: Burning; itching; foreign body sensation; tearing.

Clinical findings: Marked injection; microhemorrhages; swelling of the plicae; minimal secretion.

Unlike bacterial conjunctivitis, viral conjunctivitis is rarely related to contact lens wearing; it is usually a manifestation of systemic viral infection, for example influenza. Nonetheless, though primary viral conjunctivitis is the most common type, fitters of contact lenses must be aware that poor hygiene on their part may cause an outbreak of iatrogenic epidemic keratoconjunctivitis (EKC).

Differential diagnosis: Viral conjunctivitis is distinguished from bacterial conjunctivitis by the watery secretion in the cul-de-sac, and by the swollen plicae (particularly in EKC). Signs of infection often involve the cornea as well. Cases that fail to improve with treatment should arouse suspicion of another type of infection, such as fungal or parasitic. Foreign body reactions as well as toxic and allergic processes must be excluded.

Note: Viral conjunctivitis is highly contagious. The patient's family and acquaintances are at risk, as are the personnel and patients of the lens-fitting practice.

3. Fungal Infection

Symptoms: Foreign body sensation; eye-rubbing; sensation of heat and dryness.

Clinical findings: Marked surface injection accompanied by marked, generally livid, deep injection; whitish secretions in the cul-de-sac.

Fungal infection is rare in healthy contact lens wearers and is usually seen in those suffering from immune compromise, diabetes, or other metabolic disorders. *Candida albicans* and *Aspergillus niger* are often the cause. Fungal infections are difficult to treat. Corneal involvement or infiltration into the interior of the globe poses a major threat to vision.

Fungal infections are much more common in soft lens wearers than in hard lens wearers, as the soft lens is an ideal fungal culture medium. The organisms take the water they need from the aqueous compartment of the lens, and nutrients and electrolytes from the lacrimal fluid.

Fungal infections are best diagnosed by microbial culture of the secretions from the cul-de-sac. Microscopic examination of secretions and of the contact lens itself may reveal fungal hyphae. Demonstration of the responsible fungal organism serves to exclude other possible causes of conjunctivitis, for example GPC.

Differential diagnosis: Fungal infections of the anterior segment are not always readily distinguishable from bacterial or viral infections, particularly because mixed flora may be present. Microbial culture is required.

Prophylaxis: In general, patients at risk of fungal infection should not wear contact lenses. Those who do wear lenses must comply rigidly with the recommended lens-care routine.

Note: The diagnosis of a fungal infection in a contact lens wearer should prompt medical evaluation for latent or active diabetes or an immunocompromised state.

Focal Conjunctival Hyperemia

Focal conjunctival hyperemia is due to a spatially restricted process; thus, in contact lens wearers, it is usually found in the limbal area, (i.e., at the periphery of the contact lens). The etiology of hyperemia in contact lens wearers (as in other persons) may be toxic, allergic, metabolic, mechanical, or inflammatory.

3-O'Clock and 9-O'Clock Limbal Hyperemia

Symptoms: Increased foreign body sensation; increased tear flow.

Clinical findings: Marked dilatation of the vessels at the 3-o'clock and 9-o'clock positions. These sites are often covered with a mildly raised, yellowish deposit.

Conjunctival injection near the limbus at the 3-o'clock and 9-o'clock positions in a hard lens wearer implies an inadequate cushion of tear fluid between the lens and the eye. The lens mechanically irritates the conjunctiva and cornea during horizontal saccades. The problem may be caused by inadequate lacrimation or by poor fitting. Diagnostic assessment includes quantitative tear analysis, inspection of the sit of the lens, and slit-lamp examination of the cornea after staining.

Differential diagnosis: Conjunctival injection near the limbus can also result from local lesions of the conjunctiva and cornea.

Note: Check for corneal defects in all cases of localized conjunctival injection.

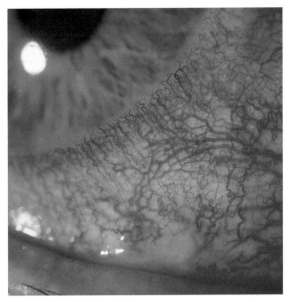

Fig. **110** Marked deep-red discoloration of the conjunctiva due to candidiasis in a soft contact lens wearer with AIDS.

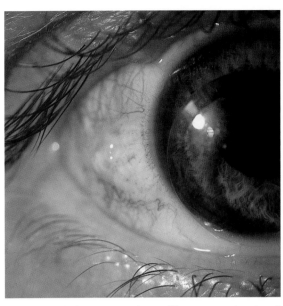

Fig. **111** Marked conjunctival vasodilatation at the 3-and 9-o'clock positions in a hyperopic wearer of hard contact lenses with tear deficiency.

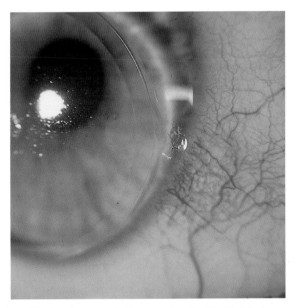

Fig. **112** Focal conjunctival hyperemia at the 4-to 5-o'clock position; injury of the edge of the cornea through improper fitting.

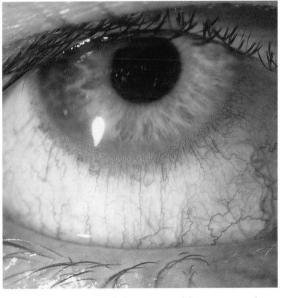

Fig. **113** Isolated perilimbal conjunctival hyperemia under a hard corneoscleral contact lens. Mechanical irritation by excessively tight fitting in the haptic zone.

Perilimbal and Limbal Injection

Symptoms: The discomfort is rarely severe and is usually limited to itching and a feeling of dryness.

Clinical findings: Markedly dilated vessels in the para-limbal or perilimbal region.

Isolated, superficial perilimbal injection is a pathological finding seen almost exclusively in wearers of soft contact lenses. It is easily mistaken for ciliary injection, which indicates an intraocular process. The affected vessels in ciliary injection are livid in color, more deeply situated, and more finely reticulated.

An arc-shaped, superficial perilimbal area of injection (sometimes accompanied by fine microhemorrhages) is usually due to faulty lens fitting. If the edge of the lens is too steep or too firmly applied to the conjunctival surface, it can compress the bulbar conjunctiva in the region of the corneal sulcus. On the other hand, if the lens is too flat, its edges can scrape the perilimbal conjunctiva. The differential diagnosis is straightforward: If the perilimbal redness disappears within 10 minutes of lens removal, the lens was too flat; if in the same period of time a reactive hyperemia appears, the lens was too steep.

Redness from wearing lenses with abrasive edges or edge defects disappears within 1–2 hours after the lenses are removed. Hyperemia of this type is only rarely associated with corneal injury.

Deep perilimbal vasodilatation indicates an entirely different situation. Deep-red or livid vessels, located below the surface and parallel to the limbus, are a definite indication of corneal damage or an intraocular process. The usual cause in contact lens wearers is toxic keratopathy in reaction either to the lens material or to a lens care product.

A finding of deep and livid (rather than superficial and brick-red) vasodilatation limited to the limbal region is classically termed "ciliary injection." The dilated vessels are located in the perilimbal sclera and are an indication of deep corneal and intraocular changes, such as iritis or uveitis, which are very rarely related to the wearing of contact lenses. It may prove difficult to determine by examination whether the finding is superficial (perilimbal) or deep (ciliary), particularly in protracted cases. A rule of thumb for the crucial differentiation of primary intraocular problems from contact lens complications is that the latter, unlike the former, generally resolve after the lenses are removed.

Table **14** Differential diagnosis of perilimbal hyperemia in contact lens wearers

Color	Location	Cause
Brick-red	Conjunctival surface	Mechanical irritation, fitting error
Bluish-red	Superficial and deep conjunctiva	Toxic, allergic reaction
Livid blue	Deep conjunctiva, sclera	Intraocular complication, iritis, iridocyclitis, uveitis

It is not always easy to classify limbal hyperemia or to determine whether it is due to the wearing of contact lenses. A thorough history and a meticulous slit-lamp examination of the limbus under highest power are mandatory. The most important criteria for differential diagnosis are listed in Table **14**.

The Ophthalmotest is an excellent aid to the examination of conjunctival changes, especially perilimbal reactions, and enables differentiation of improper lens fitting from a toxic or allergic reaction (pp. 80, 86).

Differential diagnosis: In summary, perilimbal and limbal injection must be distinguished from scleral and intraocular processes, which cause deep perilimbal (particularly ciliary) vasodilatation and thereby produce a livid (bluish-purple)—rather than brick-red—perilimbal ring.

Prophylaxis: Immediate ophthalmological examination in the early phase of perilimbal injection can prevent further injury.

Note: Intraocular disease must be ruled out whenever perilimbal vasodilatation is found.

114

115

116

117

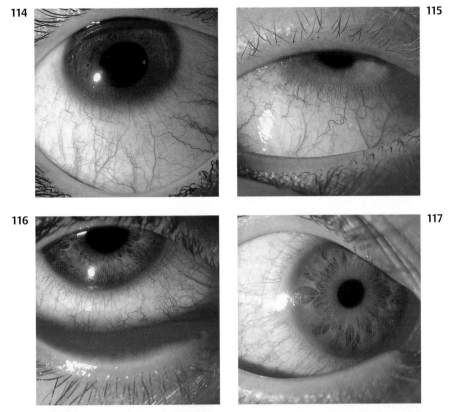

Fig. **114** Focal conjunctival hyperemia at the limbus; hard contact lens; tear deficiency.

Fig. **116** Diffuse vasodilatation of the bulbar conjunctiva with accentuation at the limbus; dry eye; gel contact lens.

Fig. **115** Marked, diffuse conjunctival hyperemia; tear deficiency; soft contact lens; marked drying of the anterior surface of the lens.

Fig. **117** Diffuse bulbar conjunctival vasodilatation with accentuation at the limbus at the area of contact of the soft contact lens; deposits on the lens surface; tear deficiency.

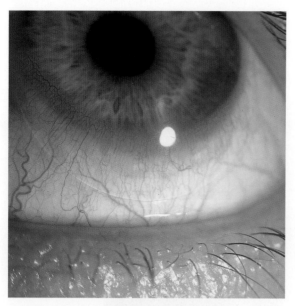

Fig. **118** Brick-red perilimbal injection from poorly seated soft contact lens; hyperopia + 6.5 D.

119

120

121

122

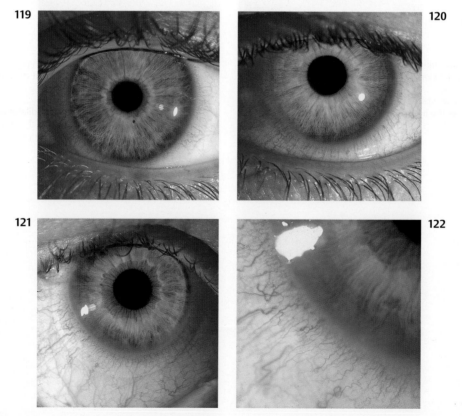

Fig. **119** Limbal hyperemia; diffuse bulbar conjunctival vasodilatation due to a toxic keratopathy; gel lenses; PMMA intolerance.

Fig. **121** Fire-red limbal hyperemia in toxic keratopathy; reaction to lens cleaning agents; gel contact lens.

Fig. **120** Limbal injection in toxic keratopathy; hyperemia of the bulbar and tarsal conjunctiva. Soft hydrophilic contact lens.

Fig. **122** Enlargement of Figure **121**.

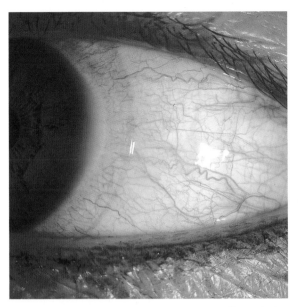

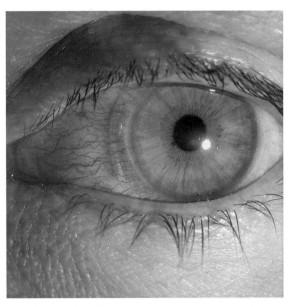

Fig. **123** Toxic conjunctival hyperemia, especially marked at the limbus, caused by PMMA allergy.

Fig. **124** Perilimbal hyperemia from toxic damage to the conjunctiva and cornea; thiomersal allergy; soft contact lens.

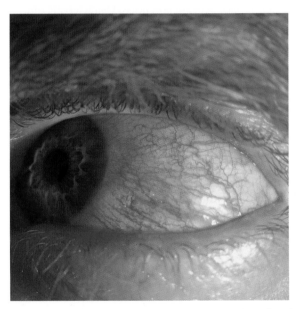

Fig. **125** Pseudoepiscleritic irritation after several weeks of wearing a defective contact lens.

Sclera

Anatomy and Physiology

The sclera, the stabilizing outer layer of the eye, is almost entirely composed of strong, interwoven, opaque collagen fibers; at the limbus, it makes a seamless transition to the transparent cornea. The sclera is completely shielded from the outside world by the conjunctiva. It is only loosely bound to the inner layer of the conjunctiva and to Tenon's capsule, with enough slack to ensure that saccadic eye movements in any direction are not hindered. Isolated pathological changes of the sclera are only rarely the result of wearing contact lenses.

Pathology

Vasodilatation and Inflammation

Symptoms: As in conjunctival inflammation: itching, foreign body sensation; rarely tearing; a sensation of pressure on the globe.

Clinical findings: Scleral vessels are a deep, livid color; concomitant conjunctival injection.

Pseudoepiscleritis can be caused by the haptic of hard or soft corneoscleral lenses rubbing against the surface of the eyeball, or by the wearing of lenses with defective edges. Vasodilatation indicates mechanical irritation or infection of the sclera; scleral infection is usually secondary to conjunctivitis or keratitis. The deep-seated, livid discoloration that typifies these scleral changes is clearly distinct from the intense, brick-red color of the overlying conjunctiva and its vessels.

> **Note:** Intraocular disease must be ruled out whenever scleral inflammation is found.

Injury and Hemorrhage

Symptoms: Foreign body sensation; pain; tearing.

Clinical findings: Hemorrhages; tissue defects in the conjunctiva and sclera.

Scleral injuries in contact lens wearers—usually bleeding cuts or small tissue defects—are usually caused by sharp or fractured contact lens edges. The overlying conjunctiva is usually involved (cut) as well. Such problems are being seen ever more frequently in wearers of disposable lenses who fail to change them as directed and are then injured by lenses that have become defective through excessive wear. Inept lens insertion or removal can also injure the sclera.

Improper sitting of either hard or soft lenses on the eye can injure the superficial scleral vessels. An unfavorable distribution of lens haptic pressure on the scleral surface beneath produces a characteristic ring of petechial hemorrhages that may coalesce to form a subconjunctival hematoma. This problem is seen less frequently at present because hard corneoscleral lenses or scleral shells are no longer fitted.

Scleral injury or inflammation is easily seen under the slit lamp, and the cause is usually easy to identify by inspecting the contact lens and checking its fit. In case of doubt, fluorescein or rose bengal can be used to highlight all tissue defects of the conjunctiva, sclera, and cornea.

Differential diagnosis: Scleral injury and inflammation can also arise from causes unrelated to wearing contact lenses. When a scleral hemorrhage is seen in a contact lens wearer, care should be taken to rule out a perforation of the globe hidden behind the hemorrhage.

Prophylaxis: Lens-related scleral injury can be prevented only by good lens hygiene and the wearing of intact lenses.

> **Note:** Whenever a scleral injury is seen, perforation of the globe and intraocular injury must be ruled out.

Cornea

Anatomy and Physiology

Most contact lens complications involve the cornea. Every contact lens covers part or all of the corneal surface of the human eye and causes chronic corneal irritation. Many different problems can result, for example, decreased wearing time and decreased visual acuity.

The corneal surface, including the tear film, is a high-quality optic surface that acts as the first (outermost) refractive medium of the eye. To provide the retina with an undistorted image, the normal cornea must maintain a tear-covered, perfectly smooth, nearly spherical front surface, an optically transparent medium, and a nearly spherical back surface.

The outer epithelial surface of the cornea is normally fully covered by tear fluid at all times. The epithelium rests upon a basal membrane and appears on slit-lamp examination as an optical void between the tear film and the more strongly reflecting stroma.

Bowman's zone lies immediately beneath the basal membrane and is intimately bound to the subjacent stroma. No internal structure of the stroma is visible under slit-lamp examination; one sees merely a fine Tyndall phenomenon with a light opalescent marbling. These findings are an optical effect rather than a feature of stromal anatomy.

The back surface of the cornea consists of a one-cell-thick layer of endothelium that is simultaneously the front of the anterior chamber. The structural and functional integrity of the endothelium are essential for regulation of corneal water content and thus corneal transparency. Endotheliopathies and keratoconus disturb this homeostatic mechanism.

The human cornea reacts to exogenous and endogenous influences—whether toxic, mechanical, or metabolic—by changing its thickness. Disruption of epithelial or endothelial function because of infection, trauma, or other pathological processes leads to an inflow of water, which rapidly binds to the stroma. Edema and reduced transparency (clouding) are the result. Corneal edema may be focal or generalized, depending on its etiology.

Adequate corneal gas exchange (O_2, CO_2), nutrient delivery, and waste-metabolite removal must be insured in contact lens wearers if corneal edema and thickening are to be prevented. The cornea obtains oxygen from the air through its front surface, by way of the tear film, from the aqueous humor through its back surface, by diffusion, and from the limbal vessels. When the eye is open, the lens-free cornea obtains most of its oxygen from the surrounding air. When the eye is closed (e.g., during sleep), oxygen enters the anterior corneal surface by diffusion from the vessels of the tarsal conjunctiva.

The wearing of contact lenses permanently interferes with this physiological mechanism by hindering tear circulation in front of the cornea. This is especially so during sleep, which explains why contact lens complications occur most frequently when the lenses are worn too long.

When a contact lens is worn, the cornea obtains oxygen from the surrounding air in two ways: by the tear-pumping effect of blinking, and by diffusion through the contact lens. Thus the oxygen permeability of the contact lens material is the most important factor in the prevention of corneal edema. Furthermore, contact lenses must be fitted loosely enough to allow uninterrupted tear fluid exchange. The tear-pumping effect works as follows: when the lids are opened, the lens is pulled upward slightly by the upper lid, causing its inferior margin to be slightly raised. Tear fluid is drawn, by capillary action, into the space thus created. With each blink, an estimated 2–3 µl of tear fluid from the lower meniscus enters the so-called tear lens between the lens and the cornea. While the eye remains open, the lens drifts slowly downward again over the cornea, the pressure under the lens increases slightly, and an equal volume of fluid is expelled. The new, freshly oxygenated fluid entering with each blink carries O_2 in, while the fluid that is expelled carries CO_2 out. A properly shaped and well-fitted hard contact lens allows exchange of up to 20% of the tear lens with each blink (the precise amount will depend on the frequency and temporal course of blinking, and on the topography of the anterior corneal surface).

Epithelial Changes

Symptoms: Burning; eye-rubbing; scratching sensation; increased glare. With large defect: Intense foreign body sensation; pain; tearing; blepharospasm.

Clinical findings: Large fluorescein-stained areas seen under the slit lamp in blue light.

Edema and Staining

Every contact lens irritates the cornea and causes a variably severe edema of the corneal epithelium that is easily seen under the slit lamp with oblique illumination. The diagnosis of (excessive) epithelial edema can be confirmed with micropachymetry or confocal corneal microscopy. The edematous epithelium appears green when stained with fluorescein and viewed under the slit lamp in cobalt-blue light.

The causes of epithelial edema are listed in Table **15**. The major causes are the usual types of metabolic, mechanical, and chemical irritation that contact lenses create on the corneal surface. The rare cases of edema occurring only minutes after contact lens insertion are due to a toxic reaction to the lens material or lens care products.

Staining of the epithelium when the lenses are removed at the end of the day is not caused by mechanical or metabolic irritation, but rather by poor fitting, in most cases. If staining is seen, the fitting parameters should be rechecked. A deficiency of tear fluid can also cause staining: in the absence of tears, dried-out soft lenses abrade the anterior corneal surface, while hard lenses rub against and injure the epithelium.

The increased water uptake of the corneal stroma results from a metabolic disturbance induced by chronic hypoxia. Like corneal neovascularization, it may also be the effect of mechanical, allergic, or toxic processes.

Increased corneal thickness is easily detected by pachymetry, which thus provides a highly sensitive indicator of the eye's ability to wear a contact lens. Mild corneal edema is usually asymptomatic, but edema with a central corneal thickness (CCT) of 575 μm or more is associated with diminished visual acuity and increased glare. Both of these problems may make it dangerous for the patient to drive in the twilight or at night.

More severe edema, such as that seen in the overwear syndrome or the tight lens syndrome (TLS), causes not only a marked increase in glare, but also markedly diminished visual acuity and diminished visual contrast.

Corneal edema of mechanical origin can be prevented by limiting the daily length of wear; edema of metabolic origin, by fitting lenses of small diameter and high oxygen permeability; edema of toxic origin, by the use of conservative-free lens care products. Wearers of disposable lenses can prevent corneal edema by changing them frequently.

Differential diagnosis: Staining may also be a sign of primary eye disease, such as glaucoma, or a physical or chemical effect independent of the wearing of contact lenses.

Prophylaxis: Contact lens wearers can largely prevent corneal edema by wearing fresh lenses, caring for them appropriately, and keeping to the recommended wearing times. The prophylactic use of artificial tears can also prevent corneal edema.

> **Note:** Corneal edema caused by contact lenses is most easily diagnosed at the end of the daily period of wear.

Stippling

After fluorescein is instilled into the lower cul-de-sac and the patient is asked to blink a few times, epithelial stippling is readily seen as a collection of fine foci of staining, each about 10–20 μm in diameter, distributed on the anterior surface of the cornea like stars in the night sky. These epithelial lesions are almost always of toxic origin, most commonly in reaction to lens materials and lens cleaning solutions. They are usually accompanied by mild perilimbal conjunctival injection.

Stippling can only be seen after several hours of lens wear, except when due to incomplete neutralization of cleaning solutions containing hydrogen peroxide, in which case it may arise minutes after insertion.

Differential diagnosis: Stippling is also seen in conjunctivitis, which results from prolonged exposure to shortwave radiation at high altitudes or from welding without a protective mask.

Prophylaxis: The use of preservative-free lens care solutions usually prevents stippling.

> **Note:** Chronic stippling can develop into chronic keratitis.

Table **15**   Causes of epithelial edema
Mechanical irritation, increased lens motility, excessive lens pressure
Metabolic disturbance, hypoxia, increase in CO_2, increase in lactate and pyruvate
Tear deficiency
Altered pH
Allergic reaction to lens or lens care system
Toxic reaction to lens or lens care system

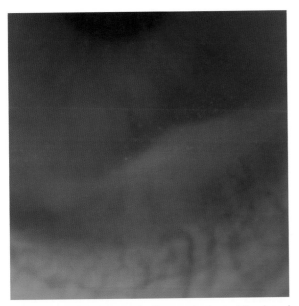

Fig. **126** Corneal staining. The fluorescein dye is diffusely and evenly distributed over the corneal epithelium.

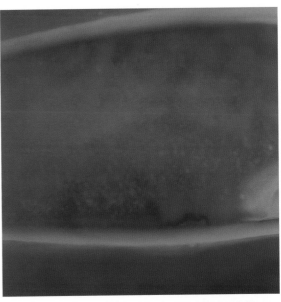

Fig. **127** Corneal stippling. Multiple stippling epithelial lesions are visible after application of a drop of fluorescein solution.

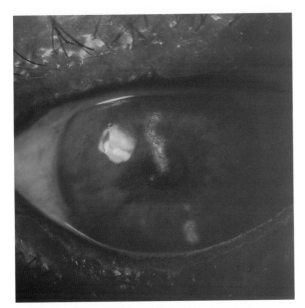

Fig. **128** Streaks and snail-like tracks in the superficial layers of the corneal epithelium.

Streaks and Spiral Traces

Streaky or spiral superficial cloudiness or opacification of the corneal epithelium is found at sites of chronic pressure on the epithelium from a soft overlying foreign body, for example, sloughed epithelial cells under the posterior surface of a hard or soft contact lens. The problem is common with poorly fitted soft corneoscleral lenses made of silicone.

Unlike corneal erosions, these areas do not stain with fluorescein, but they do stain with rose bengal. These lesions due to compression of the outermost cell layers of the epithelium may also be caused by strands of mucus collecting under lenses that have been worn for 10 hours or more. Pressure-related lesions are not easy to distinguish from the initial phase of superficial keratitis; the diagnosis can only be established by inspection of the contact lens as it sits on the cornea. Spiral traces differ from epithelial scratches and defects in that the latter always have sharp borders and stain with both fluorescein and rose bengal.

Indentations

Air bubbles between the lens and the cornea produce shallow indentations, 100–200 µm in diameter, in the outermost cell layers of the corneal epithelium. Fluorescein collects in these indentations, but the indentations themselves—unlike foreign bodies—are not stained. They resolve spontaneously within a few hours of lens removal.

Differential diagnosis: Corneal indentations can be mistaken for corneal erosions or small areas of injury due to a foreign body. Lesions of the latter types can always be stained with fluorescein; unlike corneal indentations, they retain the stain even after repeated blinking.

Prophylaxis: Corneal indentations rarely occur when contact lenses are fitted correctly and sit properly on the eye.

> **Note:** When a contact lens is fitted too steeply, air bubbles are likely to form under the center of the lens and cause corneal indentations.

Cracks

Corneal cracks are ramified, skeleton-like epithelial lesions in the peripheral portion of the cornea that stain with fluorescein and, like corneal indentations, are mechanically induced. They form under steeply fitted rigid or semi-rigid lenses and represent traces of abrasion. Though mosaic patterns in the center of the cornea (see below) develop after a few minutes of wear, cracks in the periphery, where the contact lens edges overlie the cornea, are not found till after 12–14 hours of wear. They disappear if the patient stops wearing lenses for 2–3 days.

Differential diagnosis: These lesions differ from lesions caused by foreign bodies in that the latter are sharply demarcated and do not have a ramifying, skeleton-like structure.

Spiders

Deep spider-shaped epithelial defects 50–100 µm in length are caused by proteinaceous deposits, jelly bumps, or foreign bodies on the inner surface of the lens. Movement of the lens during blinking causes abrasion of the outermost epithelial layer. The edges of the epithelial defects then become raised, and further mechanical irritation during blinking produces erosion over a wide area.

Differential diagnosis: Spider traces can be distinguished from herpes corneae by their typical branching pattern.

Mosaics

Flat-fitted, soft, hydrophilic lenses that are thick in the center, silicone lenses of older types, or large-diameter, hard corneoscleral lenses can, if worn for several hours, produce a mosaic pattern on the cornea that can be seen after fluorescein staining. A pattern like this is otherwise seen only in advanced keratoconus (the so-called Schweitzer mosaic). The corneal radii are usually flattened; pachymetric parameters are in the low normal range.

129

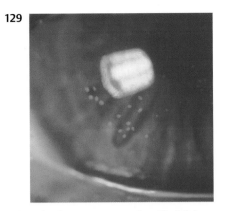

Fig. **129** Indentations in the upper corneal epithelial layer caused by persistent air bubbles in the tear film.

130

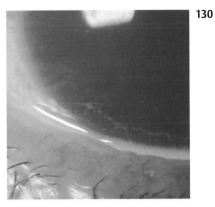

Fig. **130** Fissures indicating mechanical stress on the corneal epithelium after 12 hours of wearing a soft silicone contact lens.

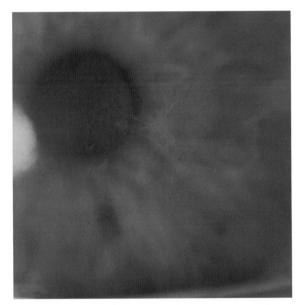

Fig. **131** Spider-shaped area of corneal epithelial clouding.

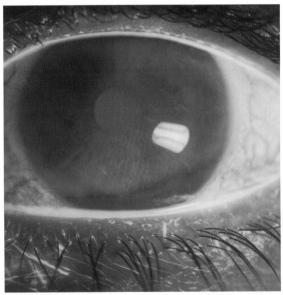

Fig. **132** Mosaic staining of the corneal epithelium after wearing a soft silicone contact lens; mechanical stress of the superficial cell layers.

The mosaic pattern is likely to be due to an electrostatic or electrodynamic effect, as these types of lens exert particularly strong frictional and shearing forces on the corneal surface. It is also thought that mosaics may be produced by pressure variations in the tear lens during blinking. Mosaics disappear several days after the lenses are discontinued and do not return when a new lens system of another type is inserted.

Differential diagnosis: Other mechanical influences on the corneal epithelium can produce mosaic figures; they can also appear spontaneously in early keratoconus, whether or not the patient wears contact lenses. Contact-lens-related mosaic patterns can be differentiated from early keratoconus by keratometry (central corneal radii of curvature less than 7.0 mm) and pachymetry (CCT less than 500 µm).

Nummules and Pseudoinfiltrates

Fine, superficial, grayish-white nummular infiltrates of the cornea may mimic epidemic keratoconjunctivitis (EKC). They appear after soft, highly hydrophilic lenses are worn for 6–12 months and are probably due to a build-up of constituents of lens-care solutions in the lens material and their subsequent release onto the cornea during lens wear.

The patient complains of gradually worsening glare, especially at night. There is no itching, burning, or pain. Unlike EKC, this form of corneal damage does not induce a reaction of the bulbar conjunctiva, and there is no swelling of the plica. The lesions heal completely, without scarring, within a few days of discontinuation of the lenses, but recur at the same site within a few days if the same lenses are reworn. Refitting with new lenses, perhaps of a different type, solves the problem. Its cause is not completely understood. Microbial cultures of the eye, lens, lens case, and lens-care products are generally sterile; chemical toxicity appears to be the etiology.

Differential diagnosis: These opacities are easily mistaken for the deeper infiltrates of EKC, nummular keratitis, and Dimmer's keratitis and can often be differentiated from them only by the minimal conjunctival and plical reaction. In this contact-lens-induced form of pseudokeratitis, unlike infectious keratoconjunctivitis, the conjunctival abnormality is usually very modest. The history and course of the problem also usually point to the diagnosis.

Prophylaxis: EKC can be prevented only by scrupulous hygiene in the lens-fitting practice.

Note: Even the suspicion of EKC in the lens-fitting practice should be taken seriously, and the strictest hygienic measures should be instituted.

133

134

135

136

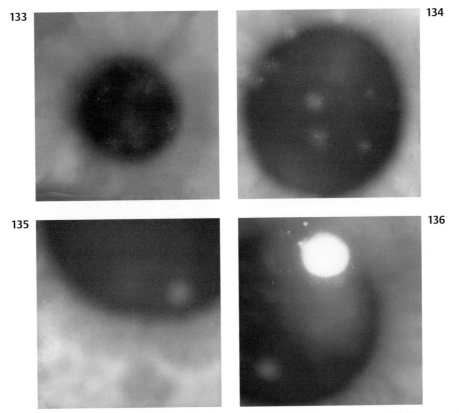

Fig. **133** Pseudokeratoconjunctivitis in a soft contact lens wearer.

Fig. **135** Pseudoinfiltrate of the cornea; sterile keratitis from silicone-lens-wear damage.

Fig. **134** Pseudokeratitis; corneal infiltrate and keratopathy after use of a quaternary ammonium-base preservative.

Fig. **136** Pseudoinfiltrate of the cornea after wearing a soft silicone contact lens.

Corneal Erosions

Symptoms: Severe, stabbing pain; blepharospasm; tearing.

Clinical findings: Corneal epithelial defects that stain with fluorescein.

Semilunar Corneal Erosions

Sharply demarcated semilunar epithelial defects are traumatic lesions caused by improper lens insertion or removal. The curved edge of the lens produces a typical arcuate injury of the outer layers of the epithelium that can extend deep into the stroma.

Platelike Epithelial Defects

Platelike defects have many causes. The cornea can be injured by improper lens insertion or removal, or by a defective lens; alternatively, corneal hypoxia in the TLS can destroy the superficial corneal epithelium. Lesions of the latter type are usually circular and located in the central portion of the cornea, while those due to mechanical injury are almost always semilunar. These differences are shown in Illustrations **1** and **2**.

Centrally located circular or oval epithelial defects are always due to hypoxia. In overwear syndrome (seen when hard or soft lenses are worn overnight), the defect is platelike and restricted to the center of the cornea because this is the area of greatest hypoxia. Unlike traumatic lesions, which always have sharp borders in the acute phase, hypoxic lesions always have indistinct borders, as can be demonstrated with fluorescein. The stroma is always swollen. These typical signs of impaired corneal metabolism are seen in overwear syndrome and in TLS, which may be considered a subtype of overwear syndrome.

Corneal erosions are painful. Lesions caused by improper lens handling always cause pain, spontaneous tearing, eye-rubbing, and a marked foreign-body sensation. In contrast, contact-lens-induced corneal hypoxia may be asymptomatic until the patient presents to the emergency department, usually in the night, complaining that the contact lens is stuck to the eye. Once the ophthalmologist has removed the lens, the damaged epithelium is exposed for the first time to the inside of the lid, and severe pain ensues, for which the ophthalmologist may be wrongly blamed.

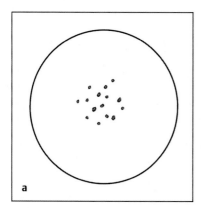
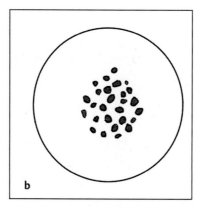
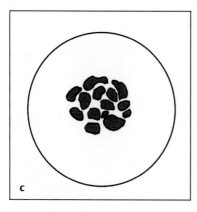
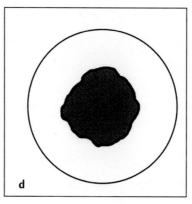

Illustration 1 Epithelial lesions due to hypoxia under a PMMA lens.

a Stage 1: after 12 hours of lens wear.
b Stage 2: after 16 hours of lens wear.
c Stage 3: after 20 hours of lens wear.
d Stage 4: after 24 hours of lens wear.

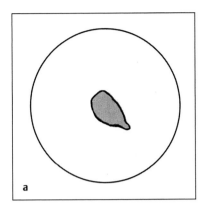

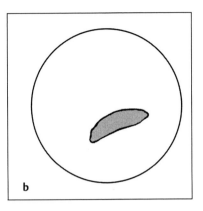

Illustration 2   Epithelial lesions of mechanical origin.

a–c Typical epithelial injuries caused by improper lens insertion.
d Pseudoherpetic lesion caused by a foreign body under the lens.
e Tracks caused by abrasion from a defective lens edge or subtarsal foreign body.
f Central round defect in overwear syndrome.

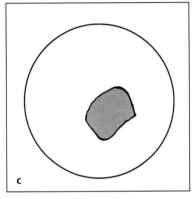

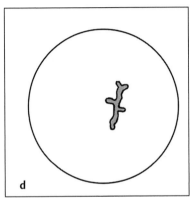

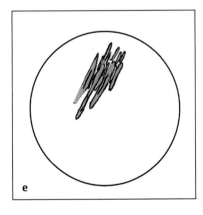

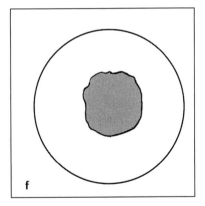

Broken-off fragments of epithelium are then found on the inside of the removed lens. Overwear syndrome is usually produced by wearing hard lenses, or soft lenses of low oxygen permeability, to bed.

Differential diagnosis: Similar lesions can be produced by exposure to full-strength hydrogen peroxide, and by ultraviolet irradiation. The differential diagnosis is made by history.

Prophylaxis: Corneal injury can be prevented only by meticulous lens insertion and removal on the part of the wearer. Overwear syndrome can be prevented by strict adherence to wearing time restrictions, including not wearing lenses during sleep. Disposable lenses, too,

should be worn no longer than recommended, as their oxygen permeability decreases significantly during wear.

Note: Only buffered eye drops or an artificial tear solution should be used when a stuck contact lens is removed. Local anesthetics are corneotoxic; they are taken up by hydrophilic lenses, and their continued presence impairs wound healing. Local anesthetics should never be used under any circumstances in the treatment of corneal epithelial lesions in contact lens wearers.

137

138

139

140

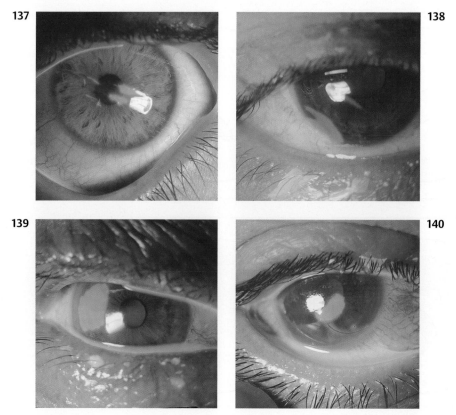

Fig. **137** Central corneal epithelial lesions after prolonged wear of a defective hard contact lens.

Fig. **138** Broad, crescentic corneal epithelial defect; typical injury due to improper insertion of a hard contact lens.

Fig. **139** Large corneal erosion after improper insertion of a soft contact lens.

Fig. **140** Central, crescentic epithelial defect caused by an eyelash trapped under a soft contact lens.

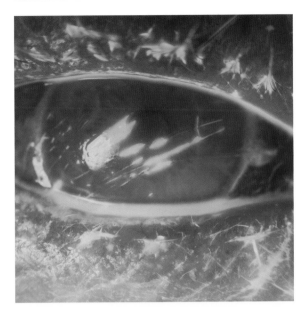

Fig. **141**   Corneal erosion; mechanical lesion; epithelial injury by a defective rigid contact lens.

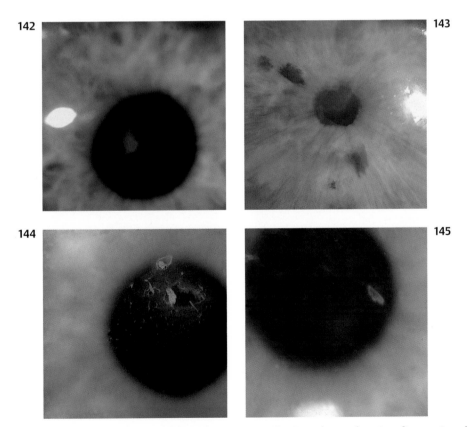

Fig. **142**   Central corneal epithelial defect and edge edema after several hours of wearing a hard, flat-fitted contact lens.

Fig. **143**   Central corneal erosion after wearing a hard lens in a dry eye.

Fig. **144**   Focal, small corneal defects under a soft lens; elevation of the epithelium at the edges; mechanical lesion.

Fig. **145**   Small, sharp-edged corneal epithelial lesion caused by defective lens material.

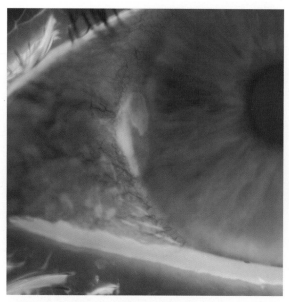

Fig. **146** Edge defect of the corneal epithelium; conjunctival injury at the 9-o'clock position caused by a flat-fitted hard lens.

147

148

149

150

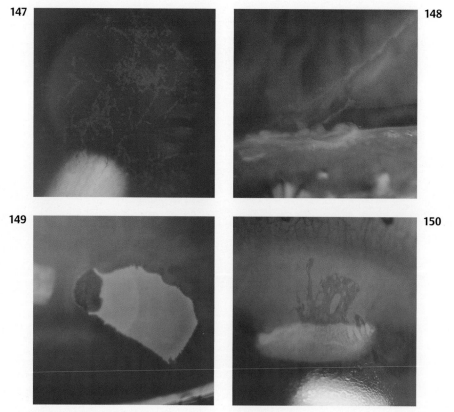

Fig. **147** Superficial, reticulated, branched corneal erosion due to a grain of sand trapped under the soft contact lens.

Fig. **149** Sharply demarcated corneal erosion; improper insertion.

Fig. **148** Corneal erosion and lid margin injury caused by the broken edge of a hard contact lens, seen after fluorescein application.

Fig. **150** Corneal tear; corneal erosion; improper insertion.

Bizarre Epithelial Defects, Branched Defects, Pseudoherpetic Defects

Streaks or deep linear grooves in the epithelium that stain with fluorescein are due to hard, sharp-edged foreign bodies between the cornea and the contact lens. The contact lens wearer fails to notice these foreign bodies before injury occurs because corneal sensitivity is reduced. Sharp-edged fractures or tears of the contact lens material can also produce deep erosions, and sometimes even cutting injuries, of the perilimbal conjunctiva and lid margins.

Such lesions can take on a variety of shapes depending on the shape and hardness of the foreign body, as well as its movement when the patient blinks. The lesions can be serpentine or branched and may resemble the lesions of dendritic keratitis.

These branched epithelial lesions are clearly of mechanical origin. If a hard foreign body with sharp edges is located between the lens and the cornea, pressure from the lens drives it into the soft corneal epithelium. With each blink, eye closure, or saccade, the lens makes a small rotatory or up-and-down movement on the surface of the eye; thus, the lesion that is created is not at a single point, but rather reflects the movements of the contact lens. Rotation of the lens usually produces a long, curved groove running parallel to the limbus, while blinking produces smaller, branched vertical defects.

Bacterial and viral cultures are of no diagnostic or therapeutic value, both because viral cultures of the conjunctival sac will occasionally be positive even in persons who do not wear contact lenses, and because the lesions will already have healed by the time the culture results are available.

Patients with a prior history of dendritic keratitis occasionally present with a clinically evident recurrence in the setting of contact lens wear. It remains unclear whether the foreign-body irritation associated with contact lens wear predisposes to such recurrences.

Differential diagnosis: Careful inspection of the inner surface of the lens reveals the causative foreign body or lens defect and thus establishes the diagnosis of a lesion of mechanical origin rather than herpes corneae; no further testing is needed. Corneal sensitivity is decreased both in herpes corneae and after long-term wearing of contact lenses, and thus is of no help in differential diagnosis. The patient's pain behavior, however, may provide a clue: herpes is painful either with or without a contact lens in place, while corneal injuries are usually not noticed until the lens is removed because the lens acts as a protective bandage.

Prophylaxis: As a rule, patients with recurrent corneal herpes should not wear contact lenses. If contact lenses must be worn, regular ophthalmological follow-up is required, particularly in the seasons of elevated risk for herpes.

> **Note:** The differential diagnosis of herpetic keratitis versus a mechanically induced corneal lesion should always be established before treatment is begun.

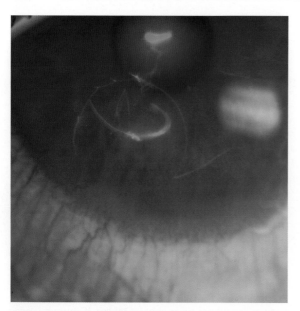

Fig. **151** Arcuate tear of the corneal epithelium caused by a defective hard contact lens.

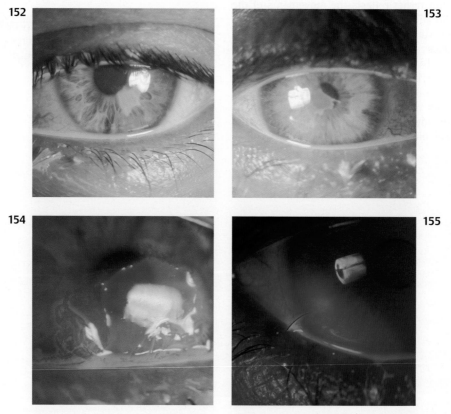

Fig. **152** Corneal epithelial defect caused by improper insertion of a hard contact lens.

Fig. **153** Corneal epithelial defect caused by improper insertion of a soft contact lens.

Fig. **154** Bubble-like corneal defect after a soft contact lens, with proteinaceous deposits on its inner surface, was worn without interruption for 40 hours; overwear syndrome.

Fig. **155** Focal corneal epithelial defect; edema due to chronic foreign body irritation (eyelash) in a wearer of hard contact lenses.

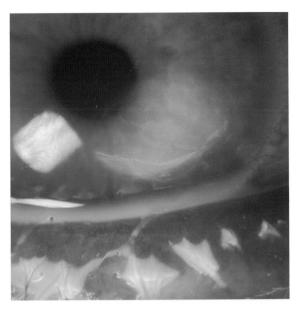

Fig. **156** Corneal tear; vesicular epithelial elevation after several hours of wearing a hard contact lens with a defective, sawtooth edge.

157

158

159

160

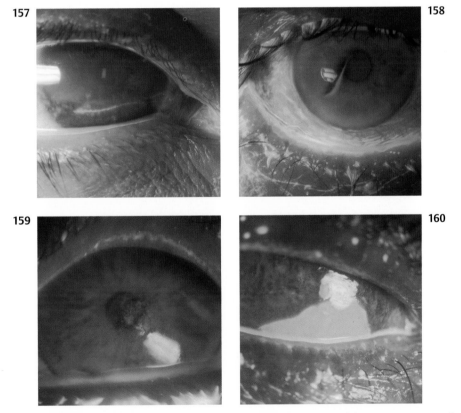

Fig. **157** Horizontal corneal lesion caused by a sharp fingernail (improper contact lens insertion).

Fig. **158** Deep corneal lesion cutting injury from the sharp edge of a lens inserter.

Fig. **159** Central, diffusely shaped epithelial defect. Peroxide injury due to faulty lens hygiene.

Fig. **160** Broad corneal epithelial defect due to accidental use of the wrong lens care product; classic severe peroxide injury.

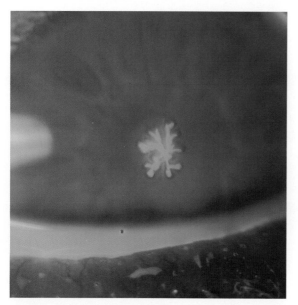

Fig. **161** Pseudoherpetic paracentral corneal epithelial defect caused by a foreign body trapped under a hard contact lens.

162

163

164

165

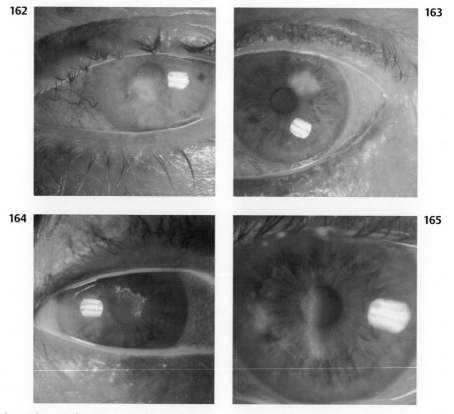

Fig. **162** Pseudometaherpetic keratitis; central corneal injury caused by a defective soft contact lens.

Fig. **164** True herpes corneae: dendritic keratitis in a soft contact lens wearer.

Fig. **163** Pseudoherpetic corneal epithelial defect; mechanical lesion.

Fig. **165** Pseudoherpetic figures in the corneal epithelium, caused by multiple grains of sand trapped under a soft contact lens.

Bubble Formation and Pseudokeratitis Bullosa

Prolonged wear of lenses that are too flatly fitted, or of soft, hydrophilic lenses that have become dirty, can cause pseudokeratitis bullosa, presumably because the lens exerts a massaging or shearing force on the cornea. This bubble-like separation of the corneal epithelium may appear even after many years of problem-free contact lens wear, perhaps in the setting of a change to a new type of lens.

Differential diagnosis: In contrast to classic bullous keratopathy, this rare contact lens complication is not accompanied by endothelial dystrophy. Stromal swelling is mild or absent, and central corneal pachymetric values are always under 650 µm.

Prophylaxis: This problem can be prevented by regular follow-up and meticulous lens hygiene. Nor should contact lens systems be changed without good reason.

> **Note:** Hard lenses that have been worn for years without problem should not be changed to soft lenses unless there is a medical indication to do so, as the change may precipitate pseudokeratitis bullosa.

Stromal Changes

Contact-lens-related pathological changes in the corneal stroma never appear in isolation, but rather always in association with changes of the epithelium and Bowman's membrane, sometimes also of Descemet's membrane and the endothelium. These accompanying changes, however, are of variable severity and may not be visible under the slit-lamp at standard magnification. Stromal defects may also be accompanied by changes in corneal topography and pachymetric values.

Edema

Symptoms: Markedly increased glare, particularly at night; decreased contrast and visual acuity.

Clinical findings: Swelling of all layers of the cornea; scattering of the slit lamp beam; elevated pachymetric values.

Stromal edema is present as an associated finding in most contact-lens-induced eye disorders, including all toxic, metabolic, and hypoxic injuries of the cornea and all lens-induced mechanical deformations of the cornea. In the latter case, the severity of stromal edema depends on the fitting technique and the lens material.

Corneal edema in contact lens wearers is of variable severity; in the early fitting stage, it is usually limited to the epithelium. Continued uptake of water causes swelling of the substantia propria and elevated pachymetric values. Pathological thickening of the center of the cornea to more than 700 µm, associated with interstitial bubble-like inclusions called "blebs," is produced by severe hypoxia.

Toxic edema regresses over weeks or months, but edema due to hypoxia or poor fitting regresses within 48 hours after the lenses are removed. Differential diagnosis is facilitated by comparative pachymetry (see pp. 109, 114, 115) of the various affected areas of the cornea. When the diagnosis is in doubt, lens wearing should be temporarily discontinued, and the corneal thickness should be measured immediately after lens removal and again 24 hours and 7 days later.

Differential diagnosis: Corneal edema also accompanies glaucoma and many other types of corneal damage, both endogenous and exogenous (e.g., ultraviolet irradiation). The diagnosis can only be established by meticulous history-taking and repeated measurement of the intraocular pressure (IOP).

Prophylaxis: Corneal edema and the glare it produces can be averted only by proper lens hygiene and compliance with the recommended maximal wearing times.

> **Note:** The IOP must be measured to rule out glaucoma in all cases of corneal edema.

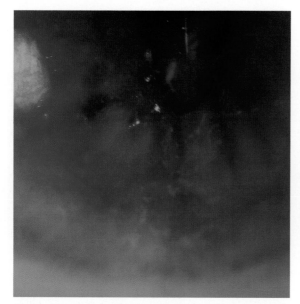

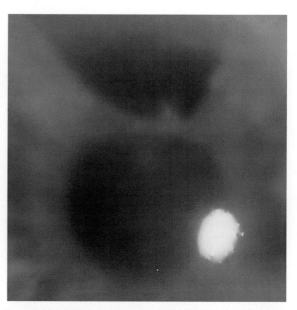

Fig. **166**   Pseudobullous keratitis after 14 years of wearing soft contact lenses.

Fig. **167**   Marked corneal edema after 96 hours of uninterrupted wearing of a soft contact lens for aphakia, unsuitable for extended wear.

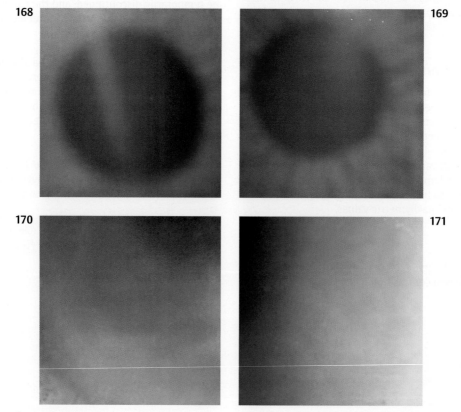

Fig. **168**   Corneal stromal edema due to hypoxia after 22 hours of uninterrupted wearing of a hard contact lens.

Fig. **169**   Corneal stromal edema due to hypoxia after 34 hours of uninterrupted wearing of a hard contact lens.

Fig. **170**   Edema affecting all corneal layers due to hypoxia after 24 hours of uninterrupted wearing of a soft contact lens.

Fig. **171**   Very severe corneal edema due to hypoxia after 48 hours of uninterrupted wearing of a soft contact lens.

172

173

174

175

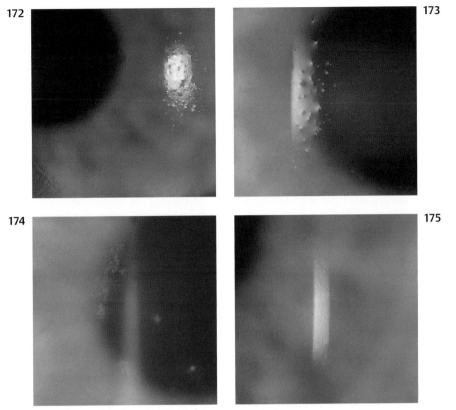

Fig. **172** Cystic corneal edema affecting all layers after a soft contact lens was worn for 48 hours.

Fig. **173** Cystic corneal edema affecting all layers after a soft, hydrophilic lens was worn for 52 hours.

Fig. **174** Cystic corneal edema affecting all layers after a hard contact lens was worn for 28 hours.

Fig. **175** Corneal edema affecting layers, with endothelial damage; chronic overwear syndrome; hard PMMA lens.

Tight Lens Syndrome

Symptoms: Severe glare; diminished visual acuity; dry-eye sensation.

Clinical findings: Very severe corneal edema; immovable, dry gel lens stuck to the corneal surface.

Tight lens syndrome (TLS) causes very severe corneal edema and is easily mistaken for an attack of acute glaucoma. It occurs exclusively after several days or, as is often the case, weeks of uninterrupted contact lens wear. Thus, it typically affects patients with extended-wear lenses who do not remove them from the eye for weeks or months at a time.

The fitting of contact lenses for extended wear has been the subject of numerous papers in recent years. Extended-wear lenses have proved their value as a refractive aid and as a therapeutic device; they have fewer complications than soft lenses that can only be worn for a restricted time each day because they do not require daily handling and cleaning. Nonetheless, extended-wear lenses are particularly fraught with the risk of TLS and other forms of severe corneal damage.

In TLS the lid margins are usually red and mildly swollen, and there is almost always a strong blepharospasm. There is marked conjunctival injection and swelling, usually more severe in the periphery than under the contact lens because of the pressure the lens exerts on the corneal surface. Once the lens is removed, however, reactive perilimbal hyperemia becomes evident within a few minutes. The cornea is swollen, blebs are frequently present, and pachymetry of the central corneal thickness yields values as high as 850 μm. In very severe and critical cases, signs of intraocular inflammation can also be seen.

If the lenses are not removed promptly, large confluent epithelial defects arise that may develop into corneal ulcers unless treatment is instituted to prevent infection. Visual acuity is reduced in all cases below the 20/100–20/200 range and is not correctable by lenses. IOP remains normal; elevated IOP suggests the alternative diagnosis of acute glaucoma.

Decreased tear flow is a very important sign of acute TLS. The Schirmer test value (with and without anesthetic) and the break-up time (BUT) are both less than half of the normal mean value for the patient's age. On retrospective review, the prefitting BUT values usually turn out to have been borderline; thus, decreased tear flow is predictive of TLS. Patients with markedly impaired lacrimation should not wear extended-wear contact lenses. Those who must wear them for therapeutic indications may suffer from chronic dryness of the eyes.

Even a mild increase in body temperature on the order of 1 °C can provoke TLS in wearers of extended-wear lenses. One reason for this is perhaps that tear flow is decreased at higher temperatures. Furthermore, measurement of upper and lower lid temperatures in patients with TLS consistently reveals an increase over baseline values, by an average of 1.5–2.0 °C. The cornea is known to consume more oxygen at higher temperatures. It is thus advisable to stop wearing contact lenses temporarily during any febrile illness, as the already subnormal amount of oxygen available to the cornea through the lens may not suffice to meet its increased metabolic requirement.

The tear fluid pH in TLS ranges from 6.8 to 7.2. It is not yet clear whether this abnormal acidity is due to excess lactic acid produced by anaerobic glycolysis, or to excess CO_2. In any case, it reflects an insufficient buffering capacity of the tear fluid.

A review of fitting data reveals that TLS is related, not only to patient-specific factors, but also to lens diameter and steepness. TLS is far more common in patients wearing lenses of diameter less than 13 mm or greater than 15 mm than in those with lenses of intermediate size; it is also far more common in patients with steeply fitted or poorly mobile lenses.

TLS is rare with minus lenses of power up to –8.0 diopter (D). It is more common when myopia is more severe and the contact lenses must be larger in diameter and thicker in their periphery; it is also more common in hyperopia and aphakia, which necessitate lenses of greater central thickness. Thus, the lens contour and the technical parameters of fitting play a decisive role in the generation of TLS.

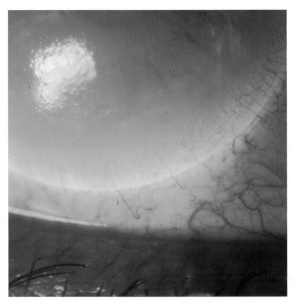

Fig. **176** Tight lens syndrome. Soft contact lens, fluorescein staining. Scattering of light at the lens surface due to desiccation (tear deficiency). Excessive corneal edema.

177

178

179

180

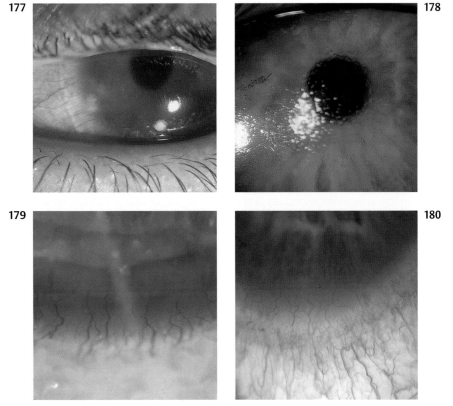

Fig. **177** TLS; marked conjunctival injection, except in the limbal area; suction effect. Dried-out soft lens *in situ.*

Fig. **179** TLS. Reactive limbal hyperemia and conjunctival edema after removal of lens. Vascularization indicates chronic corneal hypoxia.

Fig. **178** Classic TLS; dried-out surface of gel contact lens, with deposits.

Fig. **180** TLS. Limbal hemorrhage after removal of a soft lens; effect of decompression.

In acute TLS, there is a marked deposition of protein-aceous material (plaque) on the lens surfaces. Such deposits may appear over the course of a few hours, even if the patient has worn extended-wear lenses for months without any problem, in the setting of systemic changes such as a febrile illness or the use of hormone supplements or antibiotics. TLS is often precipitated by systemic illness.

Extrinsic matter (from the tear fluid or the environment) that is deposited on the surface of an extended-wear lens, or in its interior, markedly shortens the time that the lens can be safely worn. The oxygen permeability of a lens is reduced both by deposition and by aging of the hydrophilic lens material; the oxygen permeability of extended-wear lenses worn by patients who developed TLS has been shown to be only a small fraction of that of unworn lenses with the same date of manufacture.

Differential diagnosis: TLS must be distinguished from glaucoma, keratitis, and keratopathy. Thus, whenever the diagnosis of TLS is considered, the IOP should be measured and cultures should be taken.

Prophylaxis: The probability of TLS can be decreased by wearing the lenses for a shorter time each day, by not wearing them while sleeping, by applying artificial tears regularly, and by changing to rigid lenses.

> **Note:** Acute glaucoma must be ruled out in every case of suspected TLS.

Toxic Keratopathy

Symptoms: Burning; eye-rubbing; itching; increased glare.

Clinical findings: Conjunctival injection, especially in the perilimbal area; corneal edema.

Toxic keratopathy in contact lens wearers is a typical in-compatibility reaction to lens material, lens care products, or substances absorbed by the lens from the environment. Examination reveals perilimbal injection, corneal edema, and fine lesions of the corneal epithelium.

Toxic keratopathy is usually of insidious onset. After a soft contact lens is fitted, the patient notes a feeling of dryness in the eyes, which worsens over time. The eyes itch and seem to tire more rapidly; there is increased glare, particularly at night. The first objective sign, which usually appears simultaneously in both eyes, is a circle of superficial, perilimbal reddening of the conjunctiva. The abnormality always begins in the sulcal region; if the patient continues to wear the contact lenses, it extends within a few days to a week to the entire area of conjunctiva that is covered by the lens.

If the contact lenses are removed, the vasodilatation remains unchanged at first, with only minimal improvement overnight; it lasts for several days even if the lenses are not reinserted. After it has fully resolved, perilimbal injection recurs within minutes if the same lenses, or new lenses of the same type, are reinserted.

The Ophthalmotest is a useful aid to the diagnostic evaluation of conjunctival changes, especially perilimbal reactions. As shown in Illustration **3**, the test is easy to perform and determines whether the reaction is of toxic or allergic type. The test is performed when the lenses have not been worn for at least 2 weeks, 0.2 ml of a disinfectant or wetting solution is instilled into the inferior cul-de-sac. If the patient is hypersensitive to the instilled solution, a red pericorneal conjunctival ring will appear within 10 minutes.

Peroxide disinfectant solutions must be neutralized before testing; cleaning solutions must be diluted 1 : 10 with preservative-free saline to prevent false–positive responses. If lens material is to be tested, a new, unused lens should be applied, after hydration in preservative-free saline. If the lens material is the cause of the problem, a red perilimbal ring will appear within 10 minutes.

Many volatile or water-soluble substances stored in soft, hydrophilic contact lenses can induce chemosis, conjunctival hyperemia, or toxic keratopathy. Such substances can be eluted from the lens by immersion in sterile normal saline solution; the resulting eluate can be used in the Ophthalmotest. A perilimbal reaction demonstrates that the offending substance reached the eye by way of the lens (which served as a vector, but was not itself responsible for the reaction).

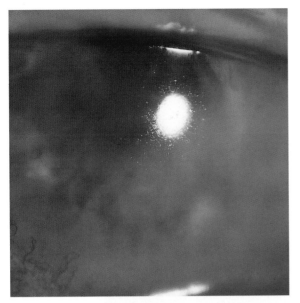

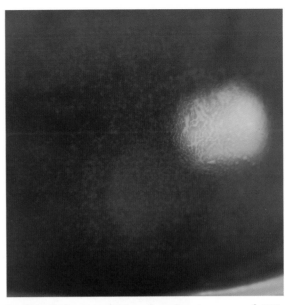

Fig. **181**   TLS; desiccated soft lens *in situ;* corneal edema, incipient vascularization. Corneal metabolic decompensation.

Fig. **182**   Toxic corneal injury from long-term use of BAC-containing lens care products with a gel contact lens.

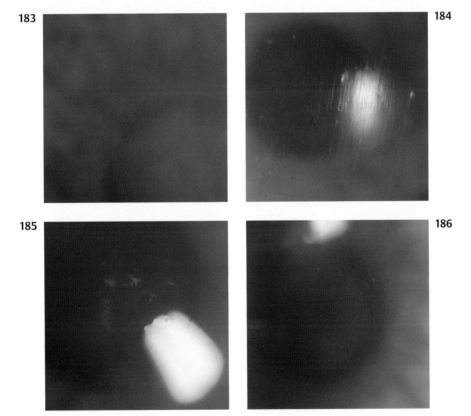

Fig. **183**   Corneal edema; epithelial defects; initial stage of a toxic reaction to a lens care agent.

Fig. **185**   Corneal edema; spider-shaped epithelial clouding; toxic reaction to BAC.

Fig. **184**   Corneal edema; vertical epithelial streaks; dry eye; toxic keratopathy due to allergy to an artificial tear solution in a soft contact lens wearer.

Fig. **186**   Corneal edema; epithelial breaks; toxic keratopathy; allergy to thiomersal and quaternary ammonium bases.

187

188

189

190

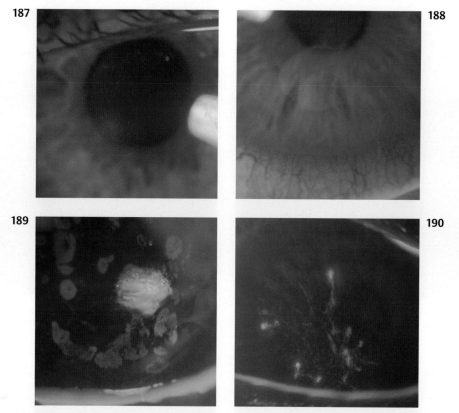

Fig. **187** Corneal edema; epithelial clouding; toxic keratopathy in reaction to chlorhexidine and thiomersal.

Fig. **189** Corneal edema and focal epithelial clouding in severe toxic keratopathy due to mixed solution syndrome (injury from lens care products).

Fig. **188** Corneal edema with superficial epithelial vesicle; peroxide injury.

Fig. **190** Corneal edema; club-shaped epithelial breaks; toxic reaction to artificial tears.

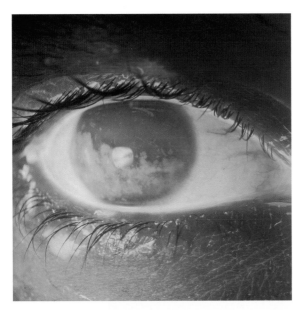

Fig. **191** Band of patchy keratopathy (reaction to preservatives).

192

193

194

195

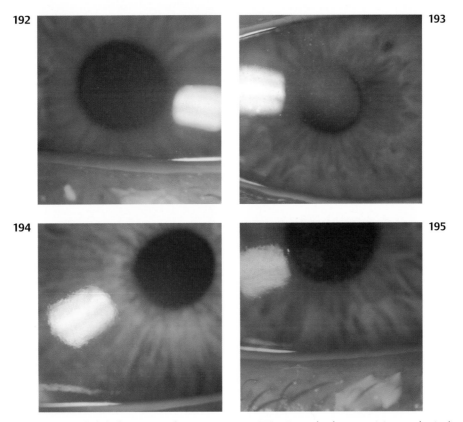

Fig. **192** Corneal edema, epithelial damage, and staining; toxic reaction to thiomersal.

Fig. **193** Corneal edema, staining, and stippling; allergy to PMMA and lens care products.

Fig. **194** Toxic corneal edema with diminished light reflex due to PMMA allergy.

Fig. **195** Toxic corneal edema with light scattering; overwear and PMMA allergy.

196

197

198

199

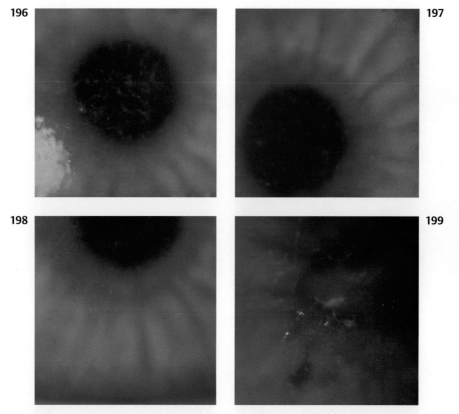

Fig. **196** Corneal edema and epithelial damage due to PMMA.

Fig. **198** Toxic keratopathy due to BAC.

Fig. **197** Toxic corneal swelling due to intolerance of a lens care product.

Fig. **199** Toxic keratopathy due to Polyquad-II.

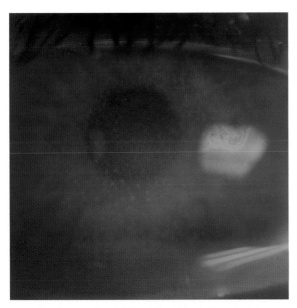

Fig. **200** Severe toxic corneal damage after years of use of astringent eye drops in combination with soft contact lenses.

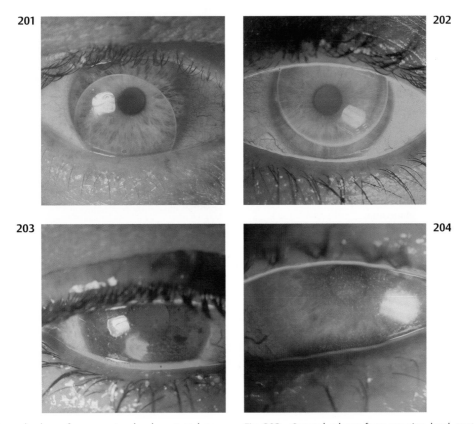

Fig. **201** Corneal edema from wearing hard contact lenses; mechanical irritation.

Fig. **202** Corneal edema from wearing hard contact lenses; metabolic disturbance.

Fig. **203** Corneal edema; epithelial defect; combined mechanical and toxic damage.

Fig. **204** Corneal edema; multiple epithelial defects in a night-sky distribution; damage due to a combination of mechanical and toxic causes (BAC).

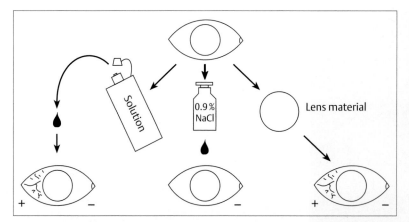

Illustration 3   Roth's Ophthalmotest. Within 10 minutes after a drop of contact lens solution is instilled into the (noninflamed) eye, marked conjunctival hyperemia develops. Preservative-free normal saline is instilled into the other eye as a control. The test may be carried out with the lens material itself or with the eluate extracted from a soft hydrophilic lens to determine the cause of allergic keratoconjunctivitis or toxic keratopathy.

The test solution just mentioned is prepared by taking the lens directly from the eye and immersing it in 1 ml of normal saline. The modified Ophthalmotest that is performed with this eluate is helpful mainly when the offending substance is suspected to be an orally or parenterally administered drug appearing in the tear fluid, or a substance entering the lens from the environment.

Differential diagnosis: Toxic keratopathy is easily confused with keratoconjunctivitis, but distinguishable from it in that the conjunctival injection seen in the latter is evenly distributed over the entire conjunctiva. Keratoconjunctivitis of viral origin is further characterized by plical swelling, sometimes even microhemorrhages. Perilimbal injection can also be a manifestation of intraocular inflammation (e.g., iritis), but in this case involves only the deeper conjunctival and scleral vessels, which appear bluish-purple, rather than bright red as in the toxic keratopathy of contact lens wearers. Whenever toxic keratopathy is suspected, the IOP should also be measured to rule out glaucoma.

Prophylaxis: Patients with a known allergic predisposition should use only preservative-free lens care products. Patients who are allergic to the lens material should change to lenses of different composition, (e.g., silicone lenses or RGP lenses), which rarely induce toxic keratopathy.

Note: When toxic keratopathy arises, the lenses should be removed and not reinserted until its cause has been determined. Toxic keratopathy can be markedly worsened by the use of a local anesthetic in the eye while the lens is still in place. In persons who do not wear contact lenses, local anesthetics in the eye are generally contraindicated as therapeutic agents, because of their high toxicity. If instilled in the eyes of patients who wear hard lenses, or (even worse) soft lenses, they can potentiate the toxicity of keratopathy-producing substances and produce irreversible corneal clouding within a few hours. Nor should a local anesthetic be used to relieve the foreign-body sensation that normally occurs when contact lenses are first fitted.

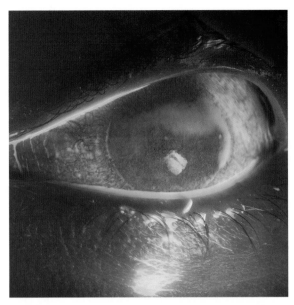

Fig. **205** Keratopathy in a bandlike distribution caused by preservatives.

206

207

208

209

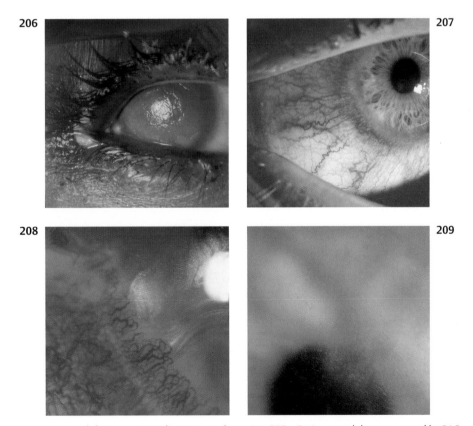

Fig. **206** Severe toxic corneal damage; peroxide injury resulting from inadvertent use instead of neutralizing solution.

Fig. **208** Toxic keratopathy caused by quaternary ammonium bases.

Fig. **207** Toxic corneal damage caused by BAC.

Fig. **209** Toxic keratopathy due to inadequate neutralization of a peroxide disinfecting solution.

Mixed Solution Syndrome

Symptoms: Severe burning; itching with eye-rubbing; tearing; marked glare; diminished visual acuity.

Clinical picture: Marked distention of the bulbar conjunctival vessels; massive, jelly-like swelling of the perilimbal conjunctiva; edema in all layers of the cornea.

A not at all uncommon complication of contact lens wearing, mixed solution syndrome is distinguishable from TLS mainly by the case history. It is clinically characterized by severe perilimbal injection and jelly-like swelling of the conjunctiva beneath a soft corneoscleral contact lens. The edema affects all layers of the cornea; pachymetry reveals a thickness at least 20% greater than normal. Fluorescein finely and diffusely stains the entire corneal epithelial surface. An Ophthalmotest performed once the problem has resolved proves that it was of toxic rather than allergic origin.

This unusually severe form of toxic keratopathy appears when multiple incompatible lens care products and/or eye drops are used in combination with a soft contact lens. The most frequent cause is adsorption onto the lens of chlorhexidine or thiomersal from one lens care product, and of a quaternary ammonium base from another. It is not clear in every instance of mixed solution syndrome precisely what compound has produced the toxic reaction, yet the problem can obviously be avoided by not using more than one lens care system for the same contact lens.

Differential diagnosis: Mixed solution syndrome should be distinguished from overwear syndrome, post-heating syndrome, glaucoma, and radiation damage (e.g., ultraviolet) of the cornea. A proper history and IOP measurement establish the differential diagnosis.

Prophylaxis: Incompatible lens care products and medications should not be used simultaneously in the eye.

> **Note:** Patients wearing contact lenses, particularly those with soft lenses, should be warned not to mix incompatible lens care products, eye drops, and artificial tears.

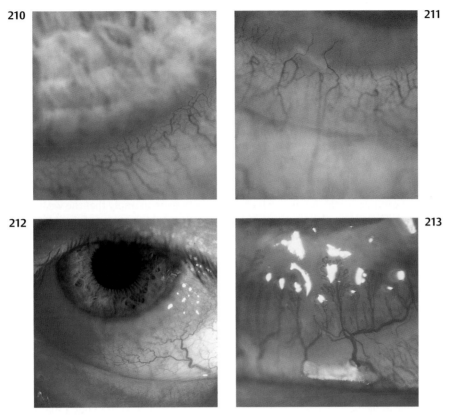

Fig. **210** Mixed solution syndrome, early stage: perilimbal hyperemia and mild corneal edema. Caused by the simultaneous use of incompatible lens care products.

Fig. **212** A severe case of classic mixed solution syndrome: massive, jelly-like swelling of the perilimbal conjunctiva, extreme hyperemia. A toxic reaction brought about by the simultaneous use of many different lens care products and eye drops for several weeks, with gel contact lenses.

Fig. **211** Mixed solution syndrome: perilimbal injection, neovascularization, corneal edema.

Fig. **213** Severe toxic keratopathy in mixed solution syndrome: perilimbal hyperemia, superficial and deep corneal vascularization, very severe corneal edema. Caused by the simultaneous use of chlorhexidine and Polyquad-II with gel contact lenses.

Corneal Deprivation Syndrome

Symptoms: Increased glare; moderately diminished visual acuity.

Clinical findings: Central diffuse clouding of the anterior stromal layers.

The first symptom of corneal deprivation syndrome (CDS) is a mild increase in glare, which then slowly progresses over several days of lens wear and finally becomes extremely unpleasant, particularly at night. Slit-lamp examination at this stage usually reveals no more than stromal edema or central corneal clouding, which is refractory to treatment. There is no obvious cause such as poor fitting, improper handling, or improper wearing of the contact lenses.

The lids and conjunctiva appear normal. The central cornea is edematous and may appear gray; higher magnification and confocal microscopy reveal subepithelial zones of cloudiness that are not characteristic of infectious, allergic, or toxic processes. These discoid zones of cloudiness lie in the anterior stromal layers, are confluent, and, unlike the classic form of lens-induced corneal edema, are found mainly in the center of the cornea. There is no abnormality of the deeper stromal layers or of the endothelium, nor are there stromal changes suggestive of hypoxia, such as blebs.

The cornea does not stain with either fluorescein or rose bengal. The pachymetric values, unlike those found in classic corneal edema, are in the high-normal range. The topographic corneal swelling quotient "Q," which enables specification of the site, origin, and extent of changes in corneal thickness or of corneal edema (see p. 114), lies between 1.0 and 1.2. Topographic study of the corneal surface reveals no deformation or sign of compression. Finally, microtopographic examination with the projection interference technique reveals only the findings usually seen in patients who wear soft contact lenses without complication.

There are no intraocular changes, and the IOP is normal. Schirmer strip values are borderline, but the BUT remains in the normal range. Visual acuity is between 20/60 and 20/100 and is not correctable with lenses.

The etiology of these changes predominantly affecting the anterior stromal layers is not fully understood. Infection is certainly not the cause: the cornea, conjunctiva, and anterior chamber are free of any sign of inflammation, and all bacterial, viral, and fungal cultures of the eye, lens, and lens case are negative. Hypoxia, too, can be excluded as a cause of CDS as it is demonstrable by pachymetry and resolves spontaneously a few hours after the lenses are removed. The absence of stromal blebs also speaks against hypoxia as the cause. The only potential contributory cause remaining in contention is a deficiency of tear flow, as all patients have Schirmer values that are on the low side of normal: Schirmer I (without anesthetic) 4–8 mm, and Schirmer II (with anesthetic) 2–6 mm.

The characteristic history and course of this syndrome seem to imply that the wearing of contact lenses has deprived the cornea of some substance, essential for its metabolic function, that it normally derives from the tear fluid. As the syndrome occurs only when the lenses are made of ionic material, one may theorize that the important substance(s) is taken up by the lens itself from the tear fluid and/or the cornea and then dropped away through the daily lens exchange, to an extent that exceeds the eye's short-term ability to replace it. In view of the chemical composition of the preionic polymers used in contact lenses, the key substance(s) must be water-soluble and present in ionized form. The deprivation hypothesis is supported by the observation that this syndrome always resolve completely after the instillation of eyedrops containing a multivitamin and multi-amino-acid preparation.

Differential diagnosis: CDS is easily told apart from corneal edema (see pp. 75, 80) by confocal slit-lamp microscopy, as well as by its course. The disappearance of discomfort and of all objective signs after two or three applications of multivitamin and multi-amino-acid eyedrops confirms the diagnosis.

Prophylaxis: Regular use of artificial tears prevents CDS; once CDS has occurred, switching to another type of lens reduces the rate of recurrence.

> **Note:** Daily disposable lenses are contraindicated in patients with decreased tear flow or metabolic disturbances affecting the cornea. When contact lenses are prescribed for medical reasons, multivitamin eye drops should be given as well.

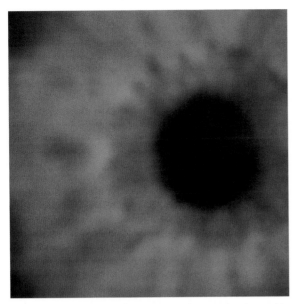

Fig. **214** CDS after several months of wearing 1-day disposable contact lenses.

215

216

217

218

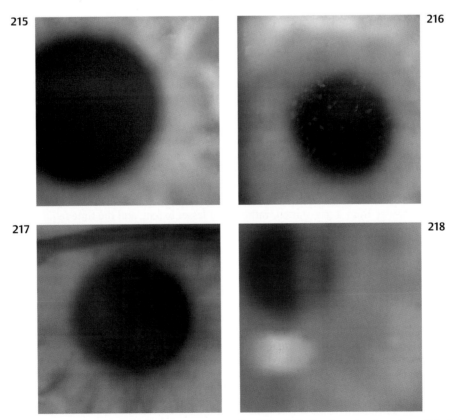

Fig. **215** CDS after 2 weeks of wearing 1-day lenses.

Fig. **217** CDS after several weeks of wearing 1-day lenses.

Fig. **216** CDS after 4 weeks of wearing soft ionic 1-day lenses.

Fig. **218** CDS after 4 months of wearing 1-day lenses made of ionic material.

Post-heat Syndrome

Symptoms: Acute, burning pain after lens insertion.

Clinical findings: Severe conjunctival injection, swelling, and cloudiness of the cornea; epithelial defects.

Post-heat syndrome, a very rare complication of wearing soft PMMA lenses, is a special type of toxic keratopathy. Its presentation resembles that of an acid or thermal burn of the cornea.

The symptoms appear immediately after a new PMMA lens is thermally disinfected for the first time and inserted into the eye. The patient complains of stabbing pain, burning, an intense foreign body sensation (symptoms closely resembling those of a corneal abrasion).

Under the slit lamp, the eye shows classic signs of an acid burn. The conjunctival vessels are dilated; in severe cases, the perilimbal vessels are paler than the vessels of the rest of the bulbar conjunctiva. The cornea is swollen; there are often diffuse epithelial defects whose blurred edges distinguish them from the sharp-edged defects seen in mechanical injury. The CCT may be 800 μm or greater.

Chemical analysis of the fluid remaining in the disinfection chamber reveals free monomers of methacrylic acid. Unless the lens is thoroughly rinsed with saline before it is inserted into the eye, residual monomers will cause toxic keratopathy.

Post-heat syndrome is clinically identical to the effect of acid or lye splashes in contact lens wearers. Patients should be instructed that this problem can also arise if they try to use household cleaning solutions (e.g., dishwashing detergent) as an inexpensive alternative to lens cleaning solutions.

We have encountered one case of ocular injury from sulfuric acid in a contact lens wearer. In an attempt to save money, the patient had mixed his own lens care solution using distilled water from a gas station, rather than from a pharmacy. Contamination with battery acid was the cause of the injury.

Differential diagnosis: These injuries are relatively rare; in suspected cases, other diagnostic possibilities include burns caused by acid, hydrogen peroxide, or ultraviolet light.

Prophylaxis: New PMMA lenses should be thermally disinfected once or twice and then rinsed in saline before insertion into the eye.

Note: Thermal disinfection has largely been replaced by cold sterilization.

Vascularization

Symptoms: Often none; in severe cases, diminished visual acuity and increased glare.

Clinical findings: Sprouting of vessels from the limbus into the cornea.

Neovascularization typically appears after months or years of wearing contact lenses. Though it has numerous causes—toxic, allergic, mechanical, and metabolic—it is thought to be most often due to the release of angiogenesis factors in response to a change in the pH of tear fluid. Neovascularization is usually most pronounced in the area underlying the upper lid and is thus easily missed on routine follow-up examination unless specifically looked for.

Soft contact lenses, especially those with large diameter or thick centers, cause neovascularization far more often than hard lenses. Thus, the periphery of the cornea should be thoroughly inspected for neovascularization in soft contact lens wearers. Ingrowth up to 2 mm beyond the limbus is acceptable, but more extensive ingrowth indicates that the cornea's physiological tolerance has been exceeded.

Neovascularization is thus an important determinant of whether hard or soft contact lenses can be worn over the long term. It should be assessed in terms of its shape, structure, extent, site, and depth. The various causes are listed in Table **16** . Branched or brushwood-like vessels appearing in the deep stroma always indicate a decreased tolerance for contact lenses, while linear surface vessels indicate a metabolic disturbance (though the etiology cannot be reliably established by the findings of slit-lamp examination alone). Pachymetry may be useful in determining the etiology of neovascularization. The central thickness of the neovascularized cornea is always elevated, to a greater or lesser extent, and the time required for it to revert to normal is dependent on the etiology: as a rule of thumb, 24 hours for edema/neovascularization due to metabolic causes, 21 days for toxic causes, and months for mechanical or postinflammatory causes.

Table **16** Causes of corneal neovascularization in contact lens wearers

Chronic hypoxia
Increased CO_2 concentration in the tear blood
Altered pH
Allergy
Toxic reaction
Chronic mechanical irritation
Postinfectious or post-traumatic scarring

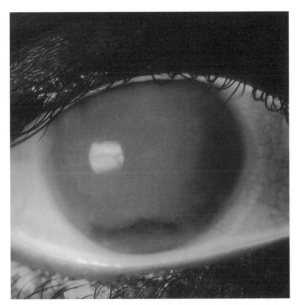

Fig. **219** Post-heat syndrome: severe toxic keratopathy after the initial wearing of thermally disinfected soft PMMA lenses.

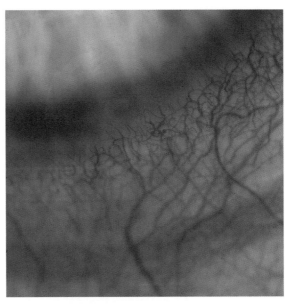

Fig. **220** Conjunctival hyperemia with incipient corneal neovascularization in a patient wearing soft lenses. Chronic conjunctivitis with mechanical irritation.

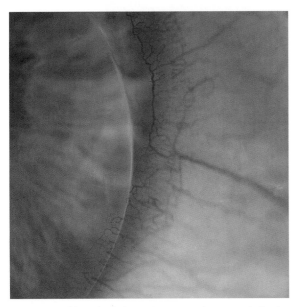

Fig. **221** Mild perilimbal injection, corneal neovascularization, formation of new vessels parallel to the limbus due to chronic hypoxia.

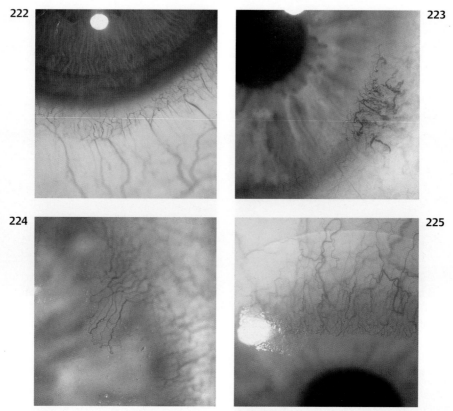

Fig. **222** Perilimbal vasodilatation, incipient corneal neovascularization, and reactive hyperemia secondary to oxygen deficiency. Steeply fitted soft lens.

Fig. **224** Limbal vasodilatation and isolated, cordlike corneal vascularization long after corneal injury by a foreign body.

Fig. **223** Local limbal hyperemia after several months of wearing a soft lens with a torn edge. Corneal neovascularization due to continuous, prolonged mechanical irritation.

Fig. **225** Limbal hyperemia in the classic 12-o'clock position under the upper lid. Combined mechanical and metabolic disturbance caused by a gel contact lens.

The site of corneal neovascularization is a further criterion in differential diagnosis. Neovascularization due to metabolic causes is usually found between the 11-o'clock and 1-o'clock positions on the limbus, where the corneal oxygen supply is lowest. Neovascularization due to toxic causes, on the other hand, is evenly distributed around the entire limbus. Ingrowth up to 2 mm is compatible with continued lens wear, as long as no progression is evident on regularly and frequently scheduled follow-up examination. If any progression is found, lens wear must be discontinued. Once the cause of neovascularization has been determined, the lens material, the fitting technique, or the lens care products must be changed, as necessary.

Deeper cuts, or infectious processes such as superficial keratitis or corneal ulceration, also frequently induce neovascularization. New vessels of this type are straight and pass radially from the limbus inward, taking the shortest route to the scarred and cloudy area of the cornea, where they branch.

Differential diagnosis: Corneal neovascularization in an otherwise asymptomatic contact lens wearer may be due to an unrelated disease process, for example a corneal laceration, burn, or abrasion, or previous corneal surgery. Neovascularization may be the first sign of graft rejection in a patient who wears contact lenses after corneal transplantation. Serial photodocumentation at frequent intervals is helpful in differential diagnosis.

Prophylaxis: Frequent follow-up examination, lenses made of highly gas-permeable material, and compliance with the recommended maximal lens wearing times lower the risk of corneal neovascularization.

Note: If contact lenses must be worn despite neovascularization, then, depending on its cause, the fitting concept should be re-evaluated or the lens material changed to another of higher gas permeability or different chemical composition. If neovascularization is thought to be partly or entirely due to a toxic reaction, the lens care products should be changed. Any degree of neovascularization into a transplanted cornea, no matter how mild, mandates immediate discontinuation of contact lenses and diagnostic assessment of the cause.

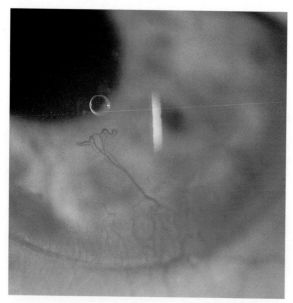

Fig. **226**   Deep linear vascularization after a corneal infiltrate.

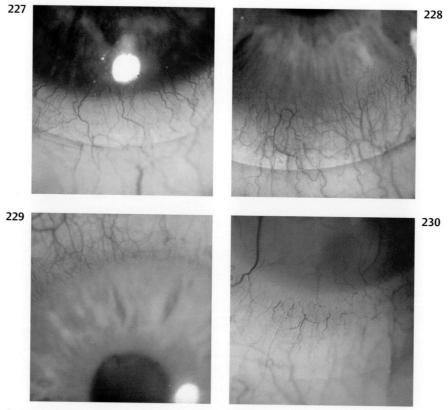

Fig. **227**   Vascularization under a soft contact lens; chronic hypoxia.

Fig. **228**   Brush-like surface vascularization and local hyperemia under a soft contact lens (metabolic disturbance).

Fig. **229**   Hyperemia under a soft contact lens; incipient corneal neovascularization; corneal edema; central epithelial defect. Chronic overwear.

Fig. **230**   Perilimbal injection; single new vessel in the cornea; marked corneal edema. Metabolic and toxic injury after several months of wearing soft contact lenses.

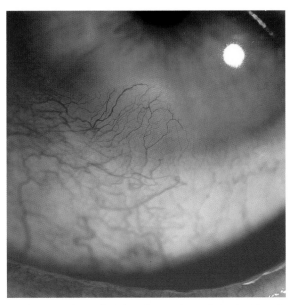

Fig. **231** Mechanically induced corneal vascularization 5 weeks after fitting of a hard contact lens.

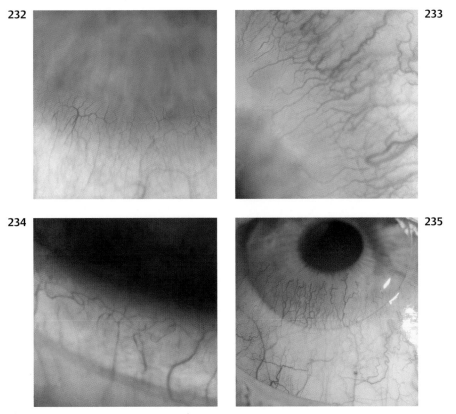

Fig. **232** Incipient corneal vascularization in a radial pattern in early toxic keratopathy.

Fig. **234** Marked hyperemia under a gel lens; incipient vascularization in toxic keratopathy (HEMA intolerance).

Fig. **233** Marked vascularization in a typical radial pattern in advanced toxic keratopathy.

Fig. **235** Marked hyperemia under the lens haptic at the 6-o'clock position; massive vascularization extending into the center of the cornea; combined metabolic and toxic corneal injury.

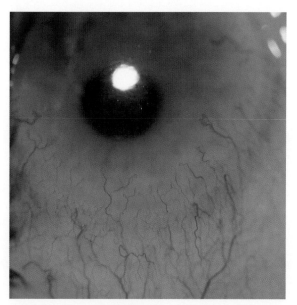

Fig. **236** Toxic keratopathy; massive neovascularization extending into the center of the cornea; corneal edema. Classic injury from lens care products.

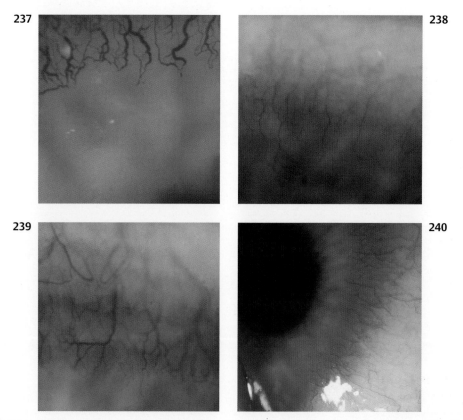

Fig. **237** Corneal vascularization and edema. Toxic keratopathy due to chronic corneal hypoxia from a soft lens.

Fig. **239** Toxic and mechanical corneal injury from a soft contact lens worn for 8 months.

Fig. **238** Superficial streaked vascularization due to a combined mechanical and toxic corneal injury from wearing a soft lens.

Fig. **240** Limbal hyperemia with conjunctival and corneal edema in toxic keratopathy caused by lens care products.

Infection

Symptoms: Burning; foreign body sensation; diminished visual acuity; increased glare; reduced visual contrast, especially at night.

Clinical findings: Conjunctival injection, especially in the perilimbal region; epithelial defects; focal clouding and swelling of the cornea, which may affect all corneal layers; deep-seated corneal processes are associated with the finding of cells in the anterior chamber.

Superficial Keratitis, Corneal Infiltrate, Corneal Ulcer

Symptoms: Foreign body sensation; tearing; eye feels hot; increased glare; diminished visual acuity.

Clinical findings: Conjunctival injection; ciliary injection; focal, punctate, grayish-white, cloudy zone of corneal edema.

Superficial keratitis, corneal infiltrates, and especially corneal ulcers are among the more serious complications of wearing contact lenses. They may cause irreversible damage, up to and including blindness due to corneal liquefaction or panophthalmitis.

Keratitis and corneal infiltrates in contact lens wearers are almost always caused by major lapses in lens hygiene or by wearing the lenses for longer than the recommended time. Inadequate lens cleaning and disinfection leads to microbial contamination. Improper insertion and removal and the wearing of old lenses that should have been discarded causes lesions of the corneal epithelium. The corneal hypesthesia of most contact lens wearers exacerbates the problem, because incipient keratitis may not produce premonitory pain that usually accompanies it.

Corneal ulcers, the most dangerous complication of wearing contact lenses, are also almost always caused by faulty hygiene on the fitter's or patient's part and are, therefore, avoidable. Corneal ulcers are usually caused by contamination of the lenses with germs such as *Pseudomonas aeruginosa* or (more recently) *Acanthamoeba*, or by exceeding the recommended wearing time. Somewhat less common causes include corneal injury from old lenses that should have been replaced, and local or global disturbance of immune defense mechanisms. The causes of corneal ulcers in contact lens wearers are listed in Table 17.

Table 17 Causes of corneal ulceration in contact lens wearers

Poor patient compliance
Faulty cleaning
Faulty disinfection
Exceeding the prescribed daily wearing time
Wearing lenses overnight or during sleep
Unhygienic surroundings
Absolute or relative tear deficiency
Hypoxia
Decreased lysozyme concentration in tears
Altered tear pH
Primary ocular disease
Tissue defects
Impaired immune competence
Environmental factors
Fever
Elevated temperature of the anterior ocular segment
Inadequate lens hygiene system
Inappropriate lens material
Altered flora
Deteriorated lenses
Increase in the corneal surface temperature

There is often an antecedent history of febrile, usually flu-like illness. Corneal ulcers can also develop when the immune system is weakened by such conditions as AIDS, leukemia, diabetes mellitus, or by antineoplastic chemotherapy.

Corneal ulcers usually occur in wearers of gel lenses and almost always affect only one eye. This is a serious condition that mandates the immediate discontinuation of contact lenses and the administration of high-dose antibiotics. Corneal scarring always develops, even if treatment is instituted promptly, and, depending on its extent and location on the corneal surface, may severely impair visual acuity. Panophthalmitis is very rare, but can occur in protracted, inadequately treated cases of corneal ulceration; it usually results in loss of the eye, which is clearly the worst complication associated with the wearing of contact lenses.

Unlike mechanical injuries to the cornea, incipient corneal ulceration is only mildly symptomatic. Pain, eye-rubbing, and a foreign-body sensation are usually well tolerated because the cornea of the contact wearer is less sensitive than normal. Patients may be disturbed only by the diminished tear flow.

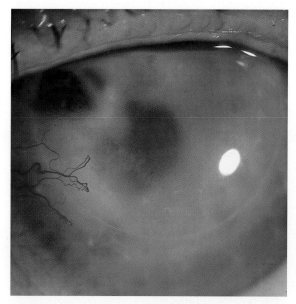 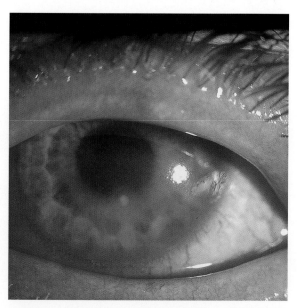

Fig. **241** Neovascularization in a transplanted cornea caused by unsupervised wearing of a soft contact lens for several months.

Fig. **242** Purulent infiltrate due to *Pseudomonas* infection under a disposable lens worn continuously for several months.

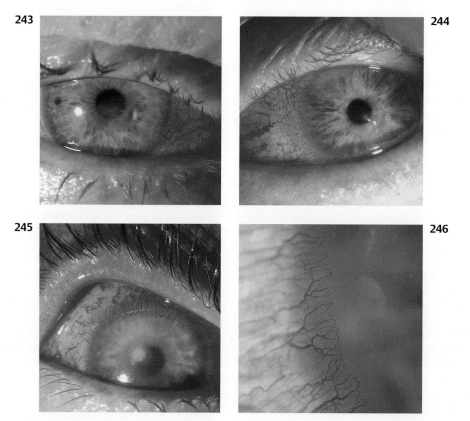

Fig. **243** Central epithelial defect and incipient ulceration with positive culture for *Pneumococcus*. Soft contact lens.

Fig. **244** Paracentral corneal ulcer with positive culture for *Staphylococcus*; improper hygiene, hard contact lens.

Fig. **245** Deep paracentral corneal ulcer with positive culture for *Pseudomonas*; overwear syndrome and faulty lens hygiene.

Fig. **246** Infiltrate in periphery of cornea; *Pneumococcus* cultured; vascularization after wearing a hard lens.

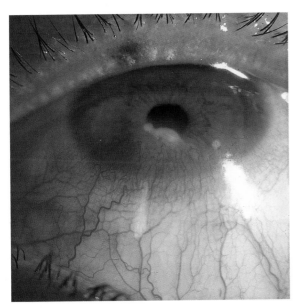

Fig. **247** Paracentral corneal infiltrate and early ulceration due to overwear of a rigid lens prescribed to treat high myopia.

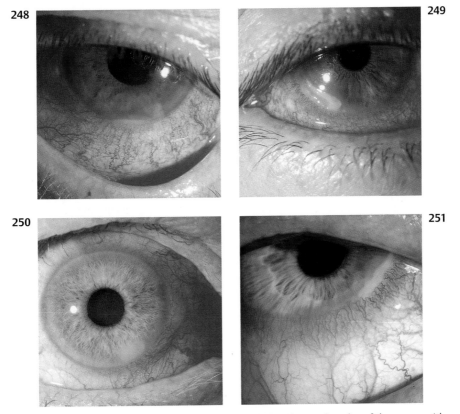

Fig. **248** Severe keratitis, early ulceration, and hypopyon after 9 months of continuous wear of a soft lens prescribed for high myopia.

Fig. **250** Peripheral corneal ulcer with positive culture for *Staphylococcus* after several months of continuous wearing of a 1-day disposable lens.

Fig. **249** Ulcer at the edge of the cornea with positive culture for *Pneumococcus* in a patient who continued to wear soft contact lenses during a febrile illness, against medical advice.

Fig. **251** Peripheral corneal ulcer after several months of continuous wearing of soft lens for aphakia.

Examination always reveals marked conjunctival injection and chemosis, with a corneal tissue defect penetrating deep into the stroma and bordered by a grayish-white, wall-like zone of infiltration. The entire cornea is swollen and the epithelium at the edge of the ulcer is occasionally raised in the form of a bleb. The anterior chamber cannot always be adequately examined under the slit lamp, but there may be a positive finding of cells and a positive Tyndall phenomenon; deep corneal ulcerations in an early phase cause fibrin to appear in the anterior chamber, and a hypopyon if they progress further, leading to a marked decline in visual acuity. The temperature of the anterior segment is increased to 1–2 °C, as is readily seen by thermography.

The microbes that most commonly cause corneal ulceration in persons wearing contact lenses are listed in Table **18**. Nearly all cases are due to *Pseudomonas*; less common are *Pyocyaneus* and fungi, the latter often in the setting of diabetes or other metabolic disorders. Recent years have seen more frequent reports of ulcers due to *Acanthamoeba,* usually from countries with a hot, arid climate, though increasingly also from the temperate zones. Thus, rinsing contact lenses with tap water should not be considered safe in any country. Corneal ulceration in contact lens wearers can also result from swimming in contaminated bodies of water.

Acanthamoeba keratitis in contact lens wearers is rare and difficult to treat. Unlike *Pseudomonas* keratitis, it usually presents with severe pain, but only minimal local findings. The fluorescein-negative subepithelial infiltrates of the initial phase sometimes have a dendritic pattern reminiscent of the infiltrates of viral keratitis, though the latter do stain with fluorescein. In fully developed *Acanthamoeba* keratitis, there is a classic ring

of cloudiness in the anterior corneal stroma, which is typically accompanied by chemosis (see p. 40), as well as perilimbal and ciliary injection of the conjunctiva.

In many cases of corneal ulceration, the causative organism can be from both the eye and the lens case. Resistance testing usually reveals that the organism is, in fact, sensitive to the particular disinfectant or hygiene system used; this implies that inadequate lens hygiene is the most important factor in the development of corneal ulcers. The rare instances of corneal ulceration becoming symptomatic in the first few days of contact lens wear are usually due to lapses in hygiene during lens fitting.

Faulty lens handling and insertion are a further cause, as corneal ulcers are more common in patients who use thermal disinfection or cold sterilization with peroxide. Lenses cleaned by the latter two methods can be recontaminated when transferred from the lens container to the eye with a dirty finger. The same can occur even with 1-day disposable lenses that are removed fresh each day from the container, as they are delivered in sterile, disinfectant- and antibiotic-free saline solution.

Microscopic examination of gel lenses worn by patients with corneal ulcers often reveals marked deposition on the lens surface, usually of proteinaceous matter or jelly bumps, which most commonly appear on highly hydrophilic soft lenses. Such deposition may be due to defects in the lens material, diminished tear secretion, or inadequate daily cleaning and disinfection, among other causes. Examination of lenses worn for long periods of time may reveal craters, surface deposits, cracks over the surfaces and on the lid margins, and polishing defects; these findings show that the lens is too old and should already have been discarded (see p. 5). Wearing such lenses traumatizes the corneal epithelium.

Some patients wear old, defective lenses despite the associated increased foreign body sensation and diminished visual acuity. The defects cause chronic mechanical irritation of the conjunctiva and cornea, which sometimes leads to permanent epithelial damage. Here microbial pathogens find fertile ground. Furthermore, the oxygen permeability (Dk) of old lenses is often only 10% that of a new lens of the same type, rendering the cornea more vulnerable to anaerobic bacterial infection.

Table **18** Microbiological findings in corneal ulcers in contact lens wearers

Pseudomonas

Pneumococcus

Staphylococcus

Haemophilus

Acanthamoeba

Candida albicans

Aspergillus niger

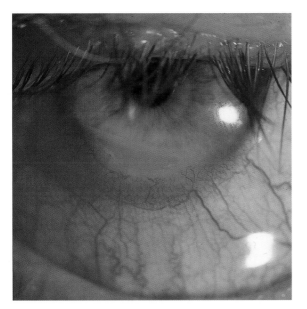

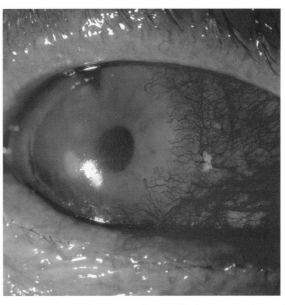

Fig. **252** Deep, crescentic corneal ulcer after continuous wearing of a hard contact lens.

Fig. **253** Severe keratitis and corneal ulceration; advanced toxic keratopathy in a soft lens wearer, after several weeks of extended wear of a non-extended-wear lens.

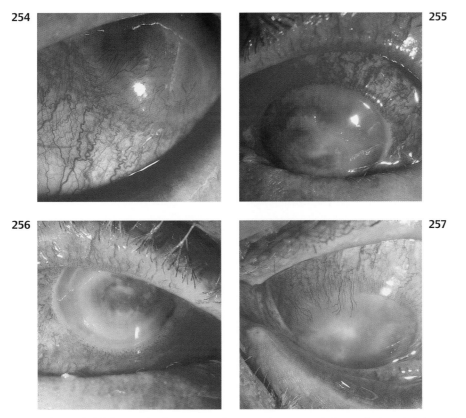

Fig. **254** Large corneal epithelial defect, early ulceration, and extensive vascularization after several months of wearing a 1-day disposable lens.

Fig. **255** Corneal ulcer with panophthalmitis from wearing a soft contact lens; severe immune compromise secondary to leukemia.

Fig. **256** Keratitis, corneal ulcer, vascularization, and panophthalmitis; mixed infection in an AIDS patient who had worn a soft contact lens.

Fig. **257** Annular corneal abscess and panophthalmitis; mixed infection in a patient with severe diabetes mellitus.

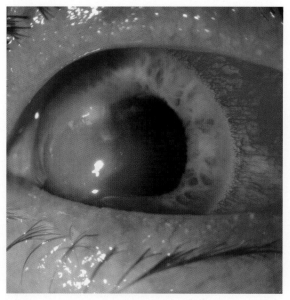
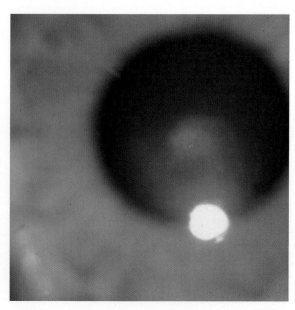

Fig. **258** *Acanthamoeba* keratitis after swimming in a quarry pond while wearing soft contact lenses; annular, grayish-white infiltrate with vesicular epithelial detachment.

Fig. **259** Central corneal clouding and incipient pseudokeratoconus after years of wearing a PMMA lens.

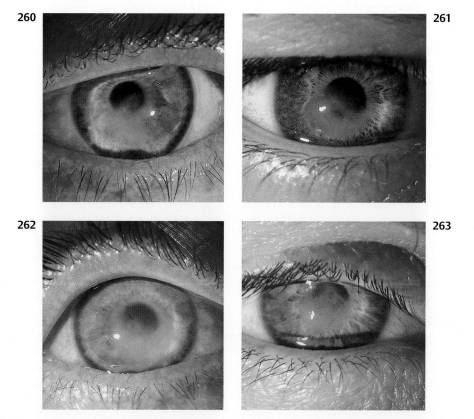

Fig. **260** Bullous pseudokeratitis caused by a flat-fitted lens.

Fig. **262** Acute keratoconus caused by wearing a flat-fitted CAB contact lens.

Fig. **261** Vesicular elevation of the corneal epithelium after wearing a soft contact lens; mechanical injury.

Fig. **263** Acute keratoconus caused by a hard PMMA lens.

Further causes of corneal ulcers include chronic mechanical irritation of the corneal epithelium by tenacious deposits on the inner surface of the lens, and elevated temperature of the anterior segment due to a fitting error impairing tear convection. Changes in tear pH alter the physiological and microbial environment of the tear fluid and the anterior segment, potentially leading to TLS, which is a possible precursor of—and the most important risk factor for—corneal ulceration.

Not only the age of the lens but also the length of time it is worn are important factors in the development of a corneal ulcer. Uninterrupted wear for 3–18 months is associated with corneal ulceration. Wearing lenses for longer than recommended frequently causes overwear or TLS; the corneal epithelial defects seen in these syndromes markedly elevate the risk of corneal ulceration. This is, indeed, the reason why patients are warned not to wear contact lenses for longer than the times recommended by fitters and manufacturers.

A case of corneal ulceration requires meticulous examination, photographic documentation, and cultures of samples taken from the conjunctiva, contact lens, and lens case, as well as of the disinfectant solution. If any culture is positive, the species should be identified and its sensitivity spectrum determined.

All patients with corneal ulcers should also be referred for a medical consultation to determine whether any form of immune system compromise is a contributing factor. The lens associated with the ulcer should be inspected under a microscope for defects or deposits, its parameters should be measured, and, if possible, its Dk should be measured and compared with that of an identical unworn lens.

Differential diagnosis: Corneal ulcers are not likely to be confused with other types of lesions, but their causation may be difficult to pinpoint and is often multifactorial.

Prophylaxis: Corneal ulcers can be prevented by meticulous lens hygiene, strict adherence to the recommended wearing times, and immediate discontinuation if a systemic infection should arise.

> **Note:** Patients with corneal ulcers should always discard their old lenses, their lens case, and any remnants of previously used lens hygiene products. They must not reinsert contact lenses until the culture of the conjunctiva is definitively reported to be negative. The use of new lenses, a new lens case, and fresh lens care products ought to prevent recontamination.

Clouding and Scars

Symptoms: No pain; diminished visual acuity; increased glare.

Clinical findings: Circumscribed, dense clouding of the cornea.

Corneal scars arise after deep traumatic injuries, such as those caused by the wearing of defective lenses; after corneal ulceration; or after many years of wearing flat-fitted hard lenses. The latter situation is the most common cause of irreversible corneal clouding in long-term wearers of contact lenses. Its typical findings include not only central corneal clouding, but also central corneal flattening and thinning of the stroma.

Central corneal clouding is a particularly common problem among patients with keratoconus and is due to excessive pressure from the fitted lens on the spherically deformed center of the cornea. The diagnosis is established by slit-lamp examination, computerized topography, and pachymetry; the latter may also help to determine the cause. Clouding of a keratoconic cornea, regardless of etiology, implies progression of disease and is a poor prognostic sign.

Differential diagnosis: The appearance of corneal scarring resembles that of corneal infection, but is distinct from it in that there is no reactive dilatation of the conjunctival and surface scleral vessels, nor is the limbal region markedly hyperemic.

Prophylaxis: Incipient corneal scarring can be detected, and its progression prevented, only by frequent follow-up of all contact lens wearers at risk.

> **Note:** Corneal scarring implies contact lens intolerance.

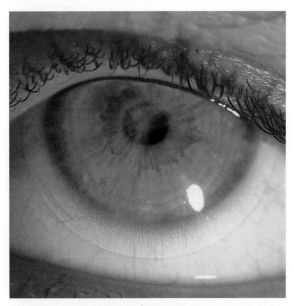

Fig. **264** Central corneal scar after 18 years of unsupervised wear of a soft hydrophilic contact lens.

265

266

267

268

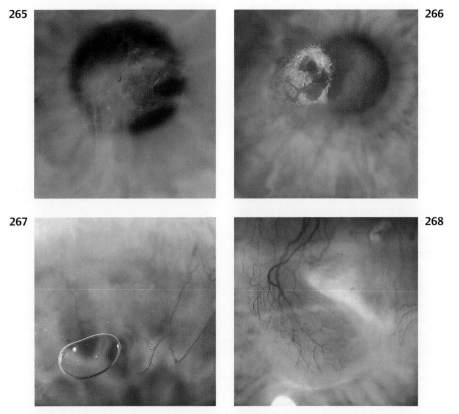

Fig. **265** Central corneal scar and stromal thinning after 33 years of wearing a hard contact lens.

Fig. **266** Central corneal scar after 34 years of wearing hard contact lenses for keratoconus.

Fig. **267** Peripheral corneal scar with vascularization and a nearby air bubble; hard contact lens, irregular astigmatism.

Fig. **268** Deep corneal scar after repeated corneal ulceration; vascularization. Hard contact lens for high myopia.

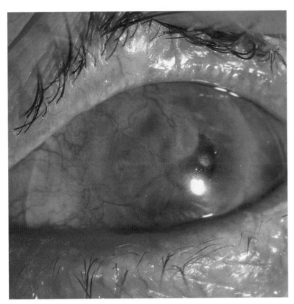

Fig. **269** Dense central and paracentral corneal scar after many years of unsupervised extended wear of a soft contact lens.

270

271

272

273

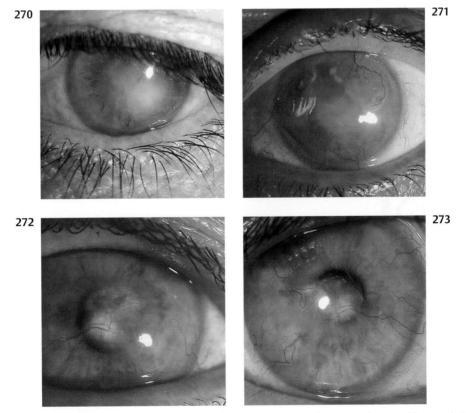

Fig. **270** Corneal leukoma after 43 years of wearing a hard PMMA contact lens for high myopia.

Fig. **272** Deep central corneal scar; vascularization. 52 years of unsupervised wearing of contact lenses of various materials. Malignant myopia.

Fig. **271** Extensive corneal scar with vascularization; hard PMMA contact lens worn for more than 40 years.

Fig. **273** Other eye of the patient depicted in Figure **272**.

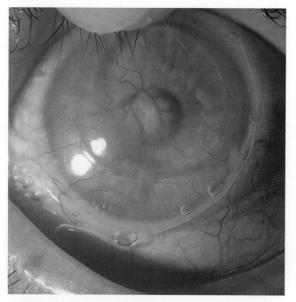

Fig. **274** Dense corneal scarring and vessel ingrowth after 56 years of wearing hard corneoscleral lenses for keratoconus.

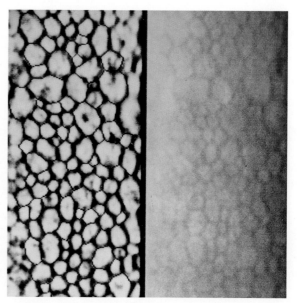

Fig. **275** Corneal endothelial changes after 10 years of wearing CAB lenses.

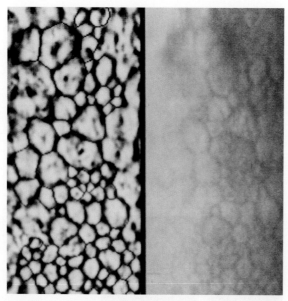

Fig. **276** Corneal endothelial changes after 30 years of wearing PMMA lenses.

Changes of Descemet's Membrane and the Endothelium

Changes of Descemet's Membrane

Symptoms: Usually none; stromal swelling causes diminished visual acuity and increased glare.

Clinical findings: Folds or tears of Descemet's membrane can be seen under the slit lamp at high power, with confocal corneal microscopy, or with the use of an endothelial lens.

Changes of Descemet's membrane, usually appearing as vertical linear streaks in the center of the cornea, are seen in keratoconus and other corneal dystrophies. Tears permit an influx of water into the stroma, which may cause worsening of the underlying condition; spontaneous tears may also be the cause of acute keratoconus where none was previously present. It remains unclear whether these changes of Descemet's membrane are due to the wearing of contact lenses; in fact, it has been maintained that contact lenses may slow, or even arrest, their progression.

Endothelial Changes

Symptoms: Mildly increased glare, usually not noticed by the patient, and occasionally halos.

Clinical findings: Marked changes in the cell count and structure; stromal swelling; increased pachymetric values.

All contact lens wearers gradually develop endothelial changes of the types listed in Table **19**. Their nature and extent depend on the lens type and mode of wear. The cell count in contact lens wearers gradually decreases over the decades, from 4000–5000/mm^2 in younger patients to 1000/mm^2 in the elderly. The cells become thin prematurely, and their shapes change. These findings may be due to chronic hypoxia, as they arise more frequently when large-diameter hard lenses or low-Dk soft lenses with thick central regions (e.g., aphakic lenses) are worn.

Table **19** Corneal endothelial changes
Diffusion disorder
Edema
Blebs
Decreased cell count
Polymegathism
Pleomorphism

Uninterrupted, extended wear of high-Dk lenses, too, can alter the cell count and cellular structure. Endothelial microscopy reveals cellular pleomorphism, along with a decrease in cell density, and polymegathism. Blebs are of uncertain significance; they are apparently associated with an increased concentration of lactic acid in the tear film, secondary to its chronically lowered oxygen concentration. The condition frequently appears in the first few months after fitting, but usually regresses thereafter.

Differential diagnosis: Corneal endothelial changes in the elderly are not necessarily pathological. Endothelial changes are the primary symptom of several types of corneal dystrophy and have also been described in advanced stages of keratoconus.

> **Note:** Endothelial changes per se do not mandate discontinuation of the contact lens but should be followed closely. Hard lenses should be discontinued if endothelial changes are found with concomitant bullous keratopathy, because there is a danger that the epithelium may be injured and become detached from the basal membrane.

Topographic Changes

Symptoms: Transient or persistent changes in visual acuity; disturbances in vision when changing from contact lenses to spectacles.

Clinical findings: Deformation of the corneal topography; change in corneal thickness; change in refraction.

High-resolution ultrasound pachymetry currently enables measurement of the corneal thickness at any point with high precision. Such measurements taken at the center and periphery of the cornea before and after a contact lens is fitted reveal that the cornea may become thicker or thinner at any point, depending on the type of lens. Flat-fitted lenses cause central thinning as an effect of direct pressure, while steep lenses cause hypoxia in the tear film and, therefore, stromal swelling.

Calculation of the swelling coefficient aids in the differential diagnosis. The corneal thickness is normally fairly constant well into old age but may fluctuate markedly as a result of systemic metabolic disease, elevated IOP, impaired lacrimation, infectious processes, and certain external influences. All of these factors affect the stability of the corneal structure and may create difficulty in obtaining an exact contact lens fit.

Contour Changes

All contact lenses, but especially hard ones, exert a light pressure on the corneal surface, which, in the long term, alters its topography. Flat lenses flatten the center of the cornea, thereby causing a decrease in myopia or an increase in hyperopia, while steep lenses do the reverse. The distribution of pressure on the corneal surface as a function of the fitting technique is shown in Illustrations **4** and **5**. At the sites of maximal pressure, the cornea is flattened and its thickness is decreased. This phenomenon is termed the "corneal distortion syndrome."

Corneal deformation explains why, after a few hours of wearing contact lenses, a patient cannot attain the former sharpness of vision on changing from lenses to spectacles. This "Sattler-veil" or "spectacle-blur" phenomenon may, for example, turn a nighttime drive home from a discothèque after changing from lenses to spectacles into a dangerous matter indeed. The effect can be measured with the Javal ophthalmometer (see Illustrations **6a, b**), as well as with microtopography (see Illustrations **7a, b**) after lens removal.

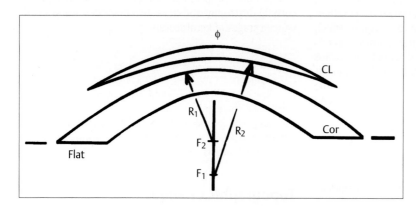

Illustration 4   The effect of pressure on the cornea from a flat-fitted lens. The radius of curvature (R_2) of the center of the posterior surface of the contact lens (CL) is greater than that of the center of the corneal surface (R_1). Prolonged wearing of a hard contact lens of this type causes flattening of the center of the cornea and elevation of its periphery. Myopia is thereby decreased.

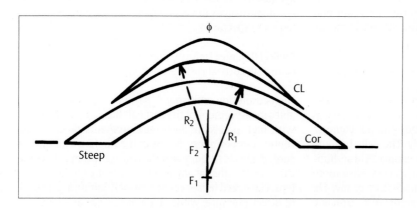

Illustration 5   The effect of pressure on the cornea from a steeply fitted lens. The radius of curvature (R_2) of the center of the posterior surface of the contact lens (CL) is less than that of the center of the corneal surface (R_1). Prolonged wearing of a hard contact lens of this type causes flattening of the periphery of the cornea and elevation of its center. Myopia is thereby increased.

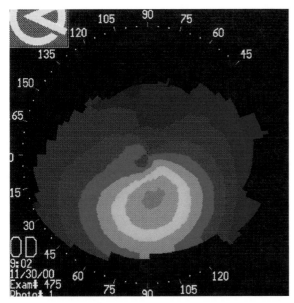

Fig. **277** Corneal topographic view after 14 hours of wearing an RGP contact lens.

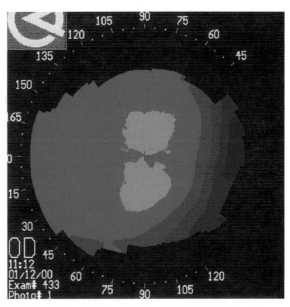

Fig. **278** Corneal topographic view after 14 days of wearing an RGP contact lens.

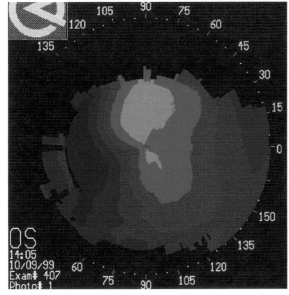

Fig. **279** Corneal topographic view after 3 months of wearing an RGP contact lens.

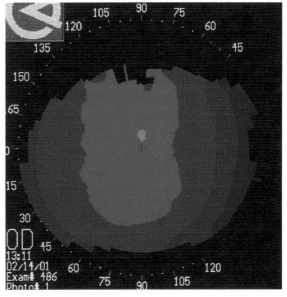

Fig. **280** Corneal topographic view after 1 year of wearing an RGP contact lens. Orthokeratologic effect.

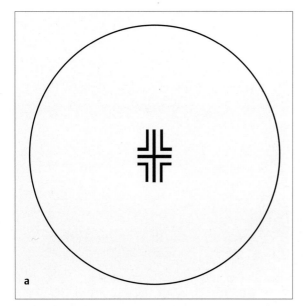 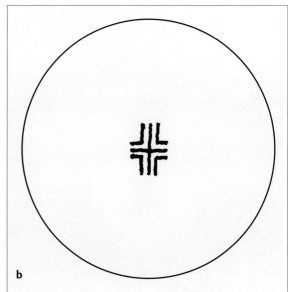

Illustration 6   Central corneal ophthalmometry/keratometry in a patient fitted with an excessively flat contact lens.
a Javal image before lens insertion.
b Javal image after 12 hours of lens wear.

Topographic changes are almost always gradual and usually regress once the patient stops wearing the lens. However, in some instances, pressure from a contact lens operating over the long term can cause irreversible irregular astigmatism or keratoconus.

In rare cases, high-grade corneal deformation occurs after only a few hours of wearing a lens because of injury to the Bowman's zone and Descemet's membrane. Central corneal thickening and steepening should arouse suspicion of contact-lens-induced acute keratoconus (in which, however, the central keratometer values are always less than 7.0 mm). Further diagnostic aid is obtained by computer-generated corneal topographic images in combination with pachymetry.

Differential diagnosis: Corneal distortion syndrome and pseudokeratoconus due to the wearing of contact lenses may either simulate or mask primary keratoconus. Pachymetry and corneal topographic imaging are the most important tools in differential diagnosis.

Prophylaxis: Long-term changes in corneal topography can be averted only by meticulous, dynamic contact lens fitting.

Note: If a transient change in refractive values is documented after the contact lenses are removed, the patient will usually not immediately regain normal clear vision with the previously prescribed spectacles. This effect must also be borne in mind when new spectacles are prescribed for a patient who will henceforth not be wearing contact lenses (for personal reasons or because of a medical contraindication). Likewise, patients who have undergone refractive surgery should stop wearing contact lenses for at least 3 months until the refractive error has stabilized and its final value can be measured.

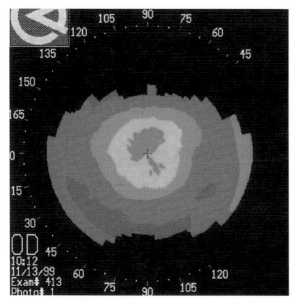

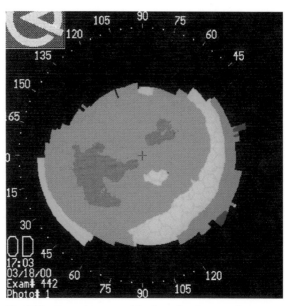

Fig. **281** Corneal topographic view after 3 months of wearing a flat-fitted RGP contact lens.

Fig. **282** Corneal topographic view after 3 years of wearing a flat-fitted RGP contact lens.

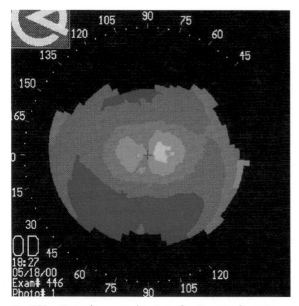

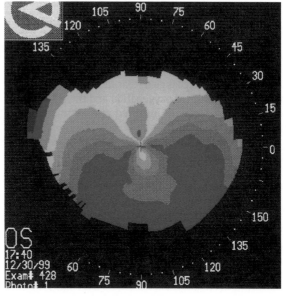

Fig. **283** Corneal topographic view after 5 years of wearing an RGP contact lens that was presumably flat-fitted. Corneal distortion syndrome.

Fig. **284** Corneal topographic view after 22 years of wearing a hard PMMA contact lens. Pseudokeratoconus.

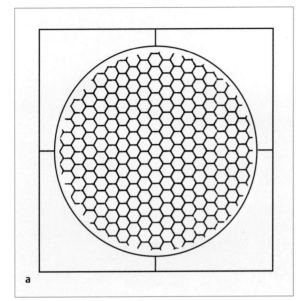 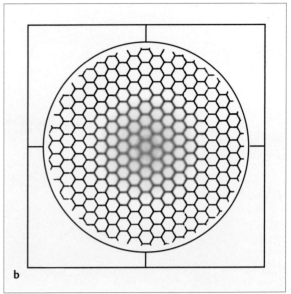

Illustration 7   Microtopography of the center of the cornea in a patient fitted with an excessively flat contact lens.
a Microtopography before lens insertion.
b Microtopography after 12 hours of lens wear.

Pachymetric Changes

Poorly fitted contact lenses cause marked changes of central and peripheral corneal thickness, which may, in turn, impair the exchange of tear fluid through convection, so that tear fluid oxygenation and the transport of metabolic products are impaired and, ultimately, corneal edema results.

The paramount role of corneal metabolism in lens-wearing comfort is readily demonstrated when experimental subjects are given lenses of varying oxygen permeability (Dk) while other parameters (thickness, shape, refractive index) are held constant. If the lens is relatively impermeable to oxygen, the CCT will increase within minutes of its insertion; if the lens is highly permeable to oxygen, it will be hours before any measurable increase in CCT is detected.

Changes in corneal thickness are also a function of the fitting technique. The CCT increases more rapidly after steep fitting than after parallel or flat fitting. Flat fitting leads to central corneal thinning with simultaneous flattening of the corneal radii, which causes transient visual disturbance when the lenses are removed.

Infectious processes and elevated IOP increase the thickness of all parts of the cornea, but contact lenses produce a difference in thickness between its center and its periphery. This differential change in thickness is quantitatively expressed as a quotient of differences in thickness, or, even better, by the swelling coefficient Q, which is defined as a quotient of swelling quotients, as follows:

$$Q = \frac{\Delta z}{\Delta p}$$

where

$$\Delta z = \frac{\text{CCT before lens fitting}}{\text{CCT after lens fitting}}$$

and

$$\Delta p = \frac{\text{peripheral corneal thickness before lens fitting}}{\text{peripheral corneal thickness after lens fitting}}$$

Here, Δz represents the change in corneal thickness at the geometric center of the cornea, and Δp represents the change in corneal thickness in its periphery, conventionally measured at a site 4.5 mm from the center. The location of this point is shown in Illustration **8**.

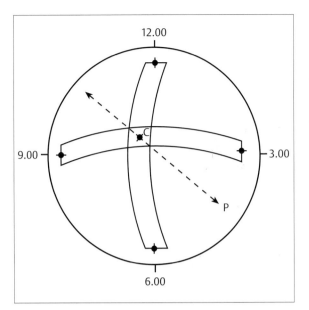

Illustration 8 The location of the points used for measurement of the corneal swelling coefficient Q. The center of the cornea is labeled C. The points P_1 through P_4 are 4.5 mm distant from C at the 3-, 6-, 9-, and 12-o'clock positions.

Q should be calculated from the measured pachymetric values each time a new hard lens is fitted. If $Q < 1$, then the lens is flat; in other words, simply stated, the lens causes the periphery to swell more rapidly than the center. If $Q > 1$, then the lens is steep, that is, there is rapid central swelling due to hypoxia. Findings of this type are reliable indicators of the steepness of fit only in the short term: all hard lenses eventually produce thinning at the corneal apex, because this area is subject to tangent forces from the mobile contact lens during blinking. Soft lenses, on the other hand, cause an increase in CCT when worn for long periods, as a result of chronic hypoxia under the center of the lens.

Inner Eye

Intraocular processes in the anterior segment are best assessed with the slit lamp, in the posterior segment with the ophthalmoscope or a contact glass. The pupils must be dilated with a mydriatic agent in either case, after removal of the contact lenses. Soft contact lenses should not be worn for at least 2 hours after the mydriasis has completely worn off; if reinserted too soon, the lenses may take up residual mydriatic agent and slowly re-release it, possibly causing pupillary disturbances for weeks afterward. Hard lenses, on the other hand, can be safely reinserted as early as 15–20 minutes after ophthalmoscopy with a mydriatic agent.

Primary intraocular diseases should be excluded before contact lenses are fitted; if any such disease is found, its severity and extent must be assessed. Not all intraocular processes interfere with the ability to wear contact lenses; for example, glaucoma, a cataract, or retinal detachment may be found in a contact lens wearer, and may worsen over the course of contact lens wear, but there is no evidence that any of these problems are exacerbated by the contact lens itself. If they arise in a contact lens wearer, they should certainly not be considered a complication of contact lens wear. The possibility nevertheless exists that long-term daily wear of contact lenses, and use of lens hygiene systems, may in fact turn out to be a contributory factor in certain types of intraocular process, even though this has not yet been found to be the case.

Longitudinal studies have shown no increased incidence of intraocular pathology in contact lens wearers compared with the general population. The rarely occurring severe complications of contact lenses, such as keratitis or corneal ulcers, can, however, be associated with secondary iritis, uveitis with or without secondary glaucoma, a complicated cataract, or (very rarely) panophthalmitis. Various possible causes of intraocular changes in contact lens wearers, without relation to contact lens wearing itself, are listed in Table **20**.

Iritis, Uveitis, Panophthalmitis

Symptoms: Pain; tearing; feeling of pressure; diminished visual acuity.

Clinical findings: The classical findings, which may be present to varying extent, include marked dilatation of the conjunctival, scleral, and ciliary vessels; cells in the anterior chamber; Tyndall effect; clouding of the vitreous humor; and elevated IOP.

Table **20**   Causes of intraocular changes in contact lens wearers

Iritis	Secondary extension of a severe infection
Cataract	Predisposition, age, exogenous and endogenous factors
Uveitis	Predisposition; secondary extension of external infection
Retinal detachment	Myopia, aphakia (not caused by wearing contact lenses)
Macular degeneration	Age, diseases unrelated to wearing contact lenses
Glaucoma	Intraocular infection, familial predisposition, age, hyperopia, hypertension

Inflammatory cells are found in the anterior chamber in iritis, iridocyclitis, and uveitis. In severe cases, fibrin or purulent material is deposited in the floor of the chamber as a hypopyon. The cornea is swollen or clouded, giving a blurred, shimmering appearance to the iris; a Tyndall effect is seen in the anterior chamber; the pupil may be deformed and attached by synechiae to the crystalline lens, and its light response may be sluggish. If secondary glaucoma develops, the IOP is usually extremely high.

If the inflammation extends from the anterior chamber into the vitreous body, it can readily develop into a panophthalmitis. Fortunately, this, the worst complication of wearing contact lenses, is extremely rare. It carries a dismal prognosis, usually ending in the loss of the eye despite high-dose antibiotic administration by whatever route (local, oral, or parenteral). The few such cases reported to date all originated from intractable corneal ulcers that caused secondary intraocular inflammation; the progression of disease was faster in cases with corneal perforation. The most common cause was infection with *Pseudomonas*, *Acanthamoeba*, or *Candida albicans*—all of which can cause particularly severe and intractable problems in immunocompromised contact lens wearers. It is thus strongly recommended that immunocompromised persons not wear contact lenses. A number of causes of diminished immune competence are listed in Table **21**.

Table **21**	Causes of impaired immune competence
Systemic infection, flu-like illness	
Postoperative state	
Diabetes mellitus	
Leukemia	
Adrenal insufficiency	
Renal insufficiency	
Pregnancy	
AIDS	
Antineoplastic chemotherapy	

Cataract

Symptoms: Gradually decreasing visual acuity and color contrast, with increased glare.

Clinical findings: Clouding of the crystalline lens.

Nowhere in the ophthalmologic literature is there any evidence of primary cataracts being caused by wearing contact lenses. This does not imply, however, that one can safely dispense with slit-lamp examination or ophthalmoscopy in the routine follow-up of the contact lens wearer. Cataracts are just as likely to develop in the older contact lens wearer as in the older wearer of spectacles. The sooner they are detected and treated in any patient, the more favorable their clinical course.

Intraocular Hypertension, Glaucoma

Symptoms: At first, asymptomatic; as the IOP rises, halos are seen at night, and the patient develops headaches, has diminished visual acuity, and sees spots before the eyes.

Clinical findings: Increased IOP; in protracted cases there are visual field defects and the optic disk is pale and excavated. If long untreated, blindness.

Untreated glaucoma predictably causes progressive visual field defects and, finally, blindness. There is no known association of glaucoma with contact lenses, but nonetheless all patients, even young patients, should be examined for glaucoma-related changes if there is any suspicion of intraocular hypertension or any family history of glaucoma. The exclusion of glaucoma should be a routine part of the follow-up examination of older patients. Contact lens wearers who complain of glare should always be examined for glaucoma, as the symptoms of glaucoma may resemble those of contact-lens-induced corneal edema, and glaucoma is easily missed in this situation if not specifically looked for.

In general, IOP should be measured after removal of the contact lens. Non-contact tonometry is somewhat less precise than applanation tonometry, but is nonetheless the preferable method in contact lens wearers. If applanation tonometry is performed, soft contact lenses should not be reinserted for at least 4 hours, or else residual fluorescein and local anesthetic in the eye may enter the lens and irreversibly stain or destroy the lens material.

Differential diagnosis: Corneal edema due to glaucoma can be erroneously attributed to another cause. The correct diagnosis can be made only by repeated measurement of IOP, examination of the fundus, and visual field testing.

Prophylaxis: The prevention of glaucoma and its consequences requires regular IOP measurement, ophthalmoscopy, and visual field testing.

> **Note:** Regular IOP measurement is mandatory in all contact lens patients over age 40 and in all patients with contact-lens-related injuries associated with a change in corneal thickness. Failure to measure the IOP in these situations is malpractice.

Retinal Diseases and Detachment

There is still no evidence for the once-prevalent notion that the wearing of large corneoscleral lenses promotes retinal detachment. This seems doubtful, in any case, as such lenses do not create any substantial mechanical stress on the eyeball. Retinal detachment is, however, a typical complication of high myopia, which is a classic indication for wearing contact lenses. Like the myopic wearer of spectacles, the myopic contact lens wearer requires frequent ophthalmoscopy to rule out retinal detachment.

Macular degeneration is similarly unrelated to contact lenses. It typically presents in the sixth or seventh decade of life with an insidious decline in central vision. Ophthalmoscopy and testing of the central visual field establish the diagnosis.

> **Note:** Like wearers of spectacles, contact lens wearers should be examined regularly for ocular diseases unrelated to the wearing of contact lenses.

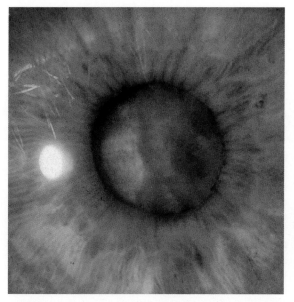

Fig. **285**   Classic senile cataract in a soft contact lens wearer; high myopia, –20 D.

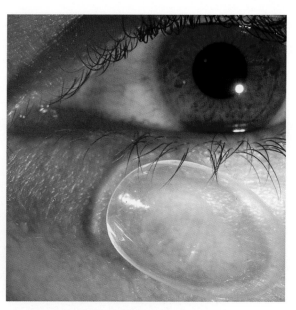

Fig. **286**   Lens loss; found attached to lower lid.

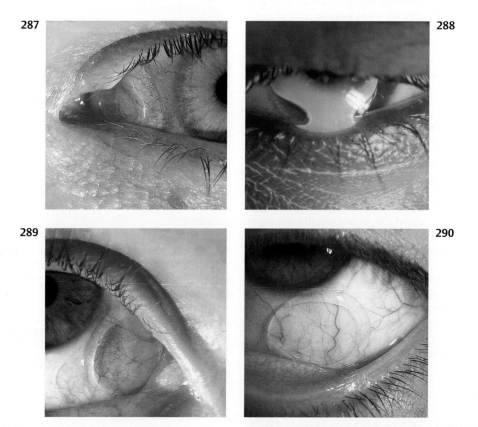

Fig. **287**   Hard lens loss; displaced to nasal canthus.

Fig. **289**   Hard contact lens displaced to the nasal canthus.

Fig. **288**   Hard contact lens in advanced keratoconus, shortly before loss of the eye.

Fig. **290**   Hard contact lens that has slipped into the lower cul-de-sac.

4 Visual Impairment

Visual Impairment

Causes of Visual Impairment

Changes in Refraction

Permanent Visual Impairment

Intermittent Visual Impairment

Glare

Causes of Glare

Diagnostic Evaluation of Visual Impairment and Glare

Visual Impairment

Some 45% of contact lens wearers complain on follow-up visits that their vision is poorer than when their lenses were first fitted; this percentage is considerably larger than with spectacle wearers. Worsened vision in contact lens wearers is usually due to faulty lens care and handling, but it may also be unrelated to the contact lenses. Contact lens wearers develop eye diseases that impair vision, such as progressive myopia, glaucoma, cataracts, and retinal detachments, just as frequently as wearers of spectacles.

As outlined in Table **22**, visual impairment in contact lens wearers can be divided into two categories. In the first category, the problem arises only when contact lenses are worn and disappears immediately when spectacles are worn instead. In the second, the problem persists when spectacles are worn.

Table **22**   Causes of visual impairment in contact lens wearers

	Findings	Cause
1. Contact lens on eye No improvement with phoropter lenses	Deposits	Material defect, tear deficiency, wetting problem, primary ocular disease
2. Contact lens on eye Improvement with phoropter lenses	Faulty insertion	Slipped or lost lens, inverted lens, lens on wrong eye, both lenses on one eye
3. Contact lens removed No improvement with phoropter lenses	Clouding of refractive media	Corneal erosion, infection, CDS, primary ocular disease
4. Contact lens removed Improvement with phoropter lenses	Orthokeratologic effect	Change in refractive error not related to the contact lens

Causes of Visual Impairment

Changes in Refraction

Faulty Lens Handling and Insertion, Lens Loss

Faulty contact lens handling and insertion can lead to visual impairment by disturbing the function of the optical system comprising the lens and the surrounding tear film. The patient may be shocked by sudden binocular visual deterioration one morning only to discover, on ophthalmological examination, that the right lens was switched with the left, or that both lenses were inserted in the same eye. Such problems are readily diagnosed with refractive testing and slit-lamp examination. Vision is immediately normalized with additional lenses in the phoropter.

If refractive testing reveals an error of 20 D or more with a rigid lens, then the lens was presumably forcibly inverted at some point during cleaning and disinfection, and thereby optically neutralized. The diagnosis can be confirmed under the slit lamp with an inverting prism or by measurement of the lens parameters.

In contact lens wearers, as in wearers of spectacles, visual impairment that is correctable with additional lenses often develops when myopia increases or decreases or when the refractive error fluctuates for other reasons. These changes are often gradual and may not be noticed by the patient until they are detected in an ophthalmological follow-up examination.

Sudden loss of a contact lens causes a marked, acute loss of visual acuity , which may be a dangerous event if, for example, the lens wearer is driving a vehicle at the time. Lens loss often occurs with vigorous movement or a blow to the head, or during water sports, where only a few splashes may suffice to wash the lens out of the eye. When the patient complains of lens loss, the examiner should verify that the lens is truly no longer in the eye, as the supposedly lost lens—or fragments thereof—is sometimes found in the conjunctival sac, occasionally weeks after the event. It may also become embedded in the conjunctival tissue and manifest itself months later as an encapsulated, chronic inflammatory process.

Permanent Visual Impairment

Primary Ocular Diseases Masked by Contact Lenses

Visual impairment caused by a primary ocular disease (e.g., clouding of the refractive media) presents in the same way in contact lens wearers as in persons who do not wear contact lenses. Determination of the cause requires testing of subjective visual acuity with and without contact lenses (or with and without spectacles, in patients who wear them).

The ocular diseases that most often impair vision in contact lens wearers are the common ophthalmological disorders: glaucoma, cataract, macular degeneration, and others. Retinal detachment occurs with equal frequency in contact lens wearers and spectacle wearers. The frequency is related to the degree of myopia, not to the wearing of contact lenses. Hyperopic eyes are prone to glaucoma. Patients with hypertension, diabetes mellitus, or other metabolic disturbances may develop chronic changes in the fundus that impair vision, whether or not contact lenses are worn.

Moreover, the contact lens wearer complaining of impaired vision should always be examined for uveitis, retinal detachment, and optic neuritis—all of which have no relation to the wearing of contact lenses, even if the patient attributes the problem to the lenses, or to the specialist who fitted them.

Thus, the treating ophthalmologist must continually bear in mind that the normal aging process, and all other disorders that can befall the eye, occur with equal frequency in contact lens wearers as in other patients. The follow-up of contact lens wearers cannot be limited to a check of the contact lens system but must also be directed toward the detection and, if possible, treatment or prevention of all such processes.

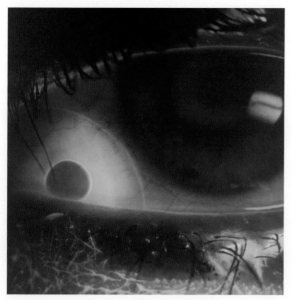

Fig. **291** "Lost" hard lens displaced into the nasal canthus; fluorescein staining.

292

293

294

295

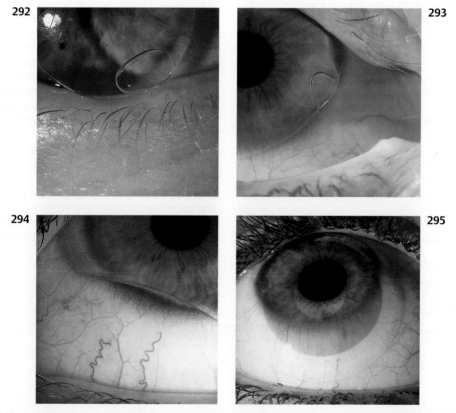

Fig. **292** Soft keratoconus lens, flatly fitted. Air bubble beneath raised edge of lens.

Fig. **294** Truncated soft toric lens, flatly fitted, superiorly displaced.

Fig. **293** Soft lens on toric cornea, flatly fitted; wrong lens type.

Fig. **295** Soft, tinted lens, flatly fitted, inferiorly displaced.

Material Defects and Defective Lenses

Visual impairment when contact lenses are worn that cannot be improved with additional lenses at the phoropter is most likely due to defective contact lenses. Possible defects include scratches, craters, fractures, deposits, and deformations (see p. 147). For example, a tear in the center of the lens causes a visual impairment that cannot be corrected with over-refraction.

The same is true of deposits, one of the commonest causes of visual problems among contact lens wearers. Lipids and proteins from the tear fluid are continually deposited on the lens surface as long as it is in the eye and will accumulate over time if the daily cleaning routine is inadequate or too infrequently performed. Jelly-bump deposits frequently form on lenses of high water content. These are stubborn calcium-protein deposits (see p. 151) that are difficult to remove and markedly impair visual acuity and wearing comfort. In most cases, the deposits cannot be removed completely and new lenses are required.

Note: Lenses with insoluble deposits or other defects should not be reworn under any circumstances, even for brief periods, because of the danger of corneal and conjunctival injury.

Intermittent Visual Impairment

Visual impairment that increases over the course of daily lens wear is due either to a fitting error or to inadequate wetting of the lens surface by tears. Patients typically report that their vision is excellent in the morning just after the lenses are inserted, but then fluctuates or deteriorates over the next few hours.

Fitting Errors

Symptoms: Good vision after insertion, but marked deterioration over the course of the day, with increased glare and decreased contrast sensitivity.

Clinical findings: Abnormal position of the lens; surface deposits; dry lens; altered corneal transparency.

Both flat-fitted and steeply fitted lenses can cause this type of problem. Very flat lenses tend to become displaced from the center of the cornea; if the lens is of high refractive power, its displacement from the center of the cornea may create an intolerable prism effect. Long-term wearing of flat lenses can also alter the corneal topography, and with it the refractive power of the eye. Such changes are easily detected by measurement of the corneal topography (see p. 110).

Excessively steep lenses may not allow adequate exchange of tear fluid; detritus collects on the lens surface, and visual acuity decreases. Improper fitting can also cause corneal edema, which manifests itself as a marked increase in glare.

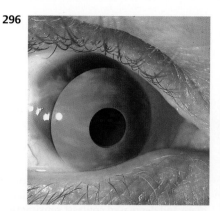

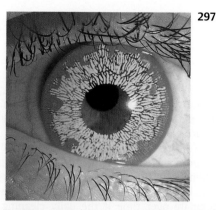

Fig. **296** Sapphire-type iris lens for traumatic aniridia. Impaired vision because of malpositioned lens of wrong type; fitting error.

Fig. **297** Painted "party lens," inferiorly displaced from the center of the cornea, causing intermittent visual impairment. Result of a car crash.

Orthokeratological Side Effects

Symptoms: Changes in refractive error and visual acuity over time as the contact lenses are worn.

Clinical findings: Different refractive power of the cornea before and after contact lenses are worn.

All contact lenses exert pressure on the center of the cornea, hard lenses more so than soft. This causes a gradual flattening or steepening of the corneal surface, while the corneal thickness may change at the same time in reaction to mechanical or metabolic irritation. These changes often impair vision in contact lens wearers. Pressure from a flat lens decreases myopia and increases hyperopia, and pressure from a steep lens does the opposite.

These orthokeratological effects manifest themselves as a difference in visual acuity between the morning state, before the lenses are inserted, and the nighttime state, after they are removed. In extreme cases, there may be a difference of several diopters. Thus, whenever patients complain of fluctuating vision of uncertain cause, it is advisable to measure the objective refractive values and the corneal radii before and after the daily period of wear, particularly in highly myopic or aphakic patients.

As the result of an orthokeratologic effect, a myopic contact lens wearer may find that his spectacles afford perfect vision in the morning, but are too strong in the evening. Occasionally, this side effect of wearing contact lenses is unethically exploited: rigid lenses can be deliberately fitted too flatly or too steeply, in order to temporarily "correct" the refractive error of the eyes to within the legally tolerated range for the issuing of a driver's or pilot's license.

Spectacle-Blur Phenomenon and Corneal Distortion Syndrome

Symptoms: When the contact lenses are removed at the end of the day, the patient is unable to regain clear vision with spectacles of any refractive power.

Clinical findings: Altered curvature of the anterior surface of the cornea.

Long-term wear of contact lenses, particularly hard lenses of low gas permeability, may lead to a worsening of the patient's vision while wearing the previously prescribed spectacles, which then does not improve when other refractive corrections are tried, whether spherical or cylindrical. This is the characteristic symptom of corneal distortion syndrome, a type of irregular astigmatism caused by the wearing of contact lenses, which is best diagnosed by computerized topographic imaging of the anterior corneal surface (see p. 110). This syndrome is also the cause of the spectacle-blur phenomenon, also known as Sattler's veil: the patient sees well with contact lenses but, on switching to spectacles, can

no longer achieve satisfactory vision, despite optimal correction. This condition creates a particular danger for the contact lens wearer who removes the lenses late at night and then tries to drive a vehicle.

The prescription of new spectacles for drivers or other patients with this problem is problematic, as the corneal topography may not return to normal for days or even weeks after the contact lenses are discontinued. In extreme cases, the irregular astigmatism is irreversible or mimics a keratoconus.

This problem is usually caused by hard, low-Dk lenses or those without aspheric geometry of their posterior surface and is rarer with the use of high-Dk rigid gas-permeable (RGP) lenses with aspheric geometry of the posterior surface. These lenses are more closely congruent with the corneal surface and alter the metabolism of the center of the cornea to a lesser extent.

Differential diagnosis: The spectacle-blur phenomenon can also be the first sign of keratoconus. The differential diagnosis can be established by computer-assisted topography of the center of the cornea.

Prophylaxis: Good contact lens fitting and the use of a gas-permeable material prevent the spectacle-blur phenomenon.

> **Note:** The spectacle-blur phenomenon is particularly dangerous when the contact lens wearer attempts to drive right after switching from contact lenses to spectacles. All contact lens wearers should be informed of this danger.

Wetting Problems

Symptoms: Fluctuations in visual acuity associated with blinking.

Clinical findings: Inadequate wetting of the lens surface; abnormal break-up time (BUT) on the lens surface.

Transient visual impairment associated with blinking implies a disturbance of wetting of the eye or of the contact lens surface. Glare is produced by cloudiness of the lens surface, the interior of the lens, or the refractive media of the eye.

Visual impairment lasting 10–20 minutes after lens insertion in the morning may also indicate a wetting problem, as tear flow is normally less during sleep. Such problems can be dealt with by instillation of artificial tears upon awakening, before the physiological inflow of tears starts. Wetting the lens after insertion may also solve the problem. Impaired vision during the day accompanied by cloudiness or glare may be a sign of early corneal edema or giant papillary conjunctivitis (GPC); these conditions are readily diagnosed with the slit lamp.

Visual impairment can result from disorders of lacrimation and the dry-eye syndrome. Any abnormality of the quality or quantity of tear fluid can impair vision in a contact lens wearer. Soft lenses need a reservoir of tears to retain their elasticity; hard lenses need a cushion of tears so that they can glide freely over the corneal surface. The tear lens between the contact lens and the cornea can only form if adequate tear fluid is present; the tear lens is an optical medium in itself and, depending on its geometry, serves as an additional plano, convex, or concave lens that cancels out small astigmatic errors. Thus, any change in the refractive index of the tear fluid, caused by fluctuations of its osmolarity, pH, or salt content, may affect visual function (cf. p. 171).

Glare

Symptoms: Increased glare, especially at night; impaired contrast sensitivity.

Clinical findings: Increased central corneal thickness (CCT), corneal edema.

Glare is an important determinant of a patient's ability to tolerate contact lenses. Glare generally increases the longer contact lenses are worn and sets a limit to the daily wearing time. Fluctuations in glare over the course of the day, in relation to wearing time and the wearing environment, are patient-specific; maximum daily wearing times cannot be prescribed according to a fixed rule, but must be individually tailored to the patient and the surroundings in which the lenses are worn.

Causes of Glare

Glare is subject to a high degree of individual fluctuation, even in persons who do not wear contact lenses, and is usually due to clouding or the refractive media of the eye (one of which is the contact lens itself). Fatigue, alcohol, drugs of abuse, and many other factors can increase glare.

Even a small amount of deposit on the surface of the contact lens, mild clouding of the lens material, or a slight change in corneal thickness can cause abnormal glare in contact lens wearers. Corneal edema increases glare and decreases contrast—problems that significantly impair sight at all times (not only when the patient drives a car at night). The causes of increased glare in contact lens wearers are listed in Table **23.** The differential diagnosis can be established by use of the slit lamp, pachymeter, and keratometer.

Prophylaxis: Because glare increases the longer the lenses are worn, patients should be advised to wear spectacles rather than contact lenses in specific situations, for example during the day if they are planning a long nighttime drive. If the contact lenses are worn at night, glare can be reduced by removing the lenses for a brief interval (1–2 hours) and cleaning them during this time.

> **Note:** Glaucoma also increases glare; it must be remembered in the differential diagnosis and excluded by measurement of the intraocular pressure (IOP).

Table **23**   Causes of glare in contact lens wearers

	Findings	Cause
1. Contact lens on eye	Deposits	Tear deficiency
2. Contact lens removed Examination immediately after removal of lens	Corneal epithelial defects	Stippling, staining, edema, corneal distortion syndrome, clouding of the refractive media, primary ocular disease
3. Contact lens removed Examination after lens-free interval of 3 days	Orthokeratologic effect	Disease unrelated to contact lens, such as cataract, glaucoma, macular degeneration, retinal detachment

Diagnostic Evaluation of Visual Impairment and Glare

The tests to be applied in the differential diagnosis of visual impairment and glare in contact lens wearers are listed in Tables **24** and **25**. These include slit-lamp examination with the lens on the eye, objective and subjective refraction with and without the lens on the eye, and careful inspection of the lenses for defects, deposits, and deformations. The corneal topography can be examined with a keratometer or ophthalmometer, or, preferably, with computer-assisted topographic imaging. The latter can be used to document changes of the anterior corneal contour over time.

If a qualitative or quantitative abnormality of the tear film is suspected, the simplest diagnostic method is the test instillation of artificial tears; if the symptoms resolve, the test provides not only the diagnosis, but also an effective treatment. If not, it may be necessary to discontinue the contact lenses for a time, and then refit them. Before refitting, however, primary and secondary ocular disorders that are unrelated to contact lens wearing must be excluded by specific testing, including IOP measurement and inspection of the anterior and posterior segments of the eye.

Note: Visual impairment of uncertain cause in a contact lens wearer requires meticulous diagnostic assessment. The contact lenses should be discontinued until the diagnosis is established, not least because wearing them may increase the risk of accidental injury.

Table **24**   Visual impairment correctible with lenses (contact lens on eye)

Cause	Diagnostic tests
Physiological fluctuation	Subjective and objective refraction
Tear film instability	Schirmer test, BUT, meniscus test, pachymetry, test instillation of artificial tears
Orthokeratologic effect	Ophthalmometry, objective refraction
Lens on wrong eye	Refraction with lens: One eye overcorrected, one eye undercorrected
Change in refractive error	Refraction determination without lens

Table **25**   Diagnostic evaluation of visual impairment of unknown origin in a contact lens wearer (no improvement with over-refraction)

Cause	Diagnostic tests
Corneal edema	Slit lamp, pachymetry
Corneal distortion syndrome	Ophthalmometry, keratometry, pachymetry
Primary ocular disease	Comprehensive ophthalmologic work-up
Contact lens deposits	Inspection of contact lenses, laboratory testing
Change in lens parameters	Inspection of contact lenses, laboratory testing

5 Causes of Contact Lens Damage

Handling, Hygiene, Wearing Times

The Patient's Hands

The Lens Case

Wearing Times

Fitting Errors

The causes of contact-lens-related ocular injury are often not immediately obvious, and their determination may take several days or even weeks. Yet a diagnosis is urgently required in every case, because nearly all patients will want to continue wearing contact lenses. Contact lenses that have been damaged in the various ways described in this chapter are a common cause of ocular injury.

Handling, Hygiene, Wearing Times

Contact lens damage is usually due to faulty lens handling and hygiene. Patients must be advised of the need to clean and disinfect the lenses regularly. Serious infections of the conjunctiva and cornea are often caused by microbial pathogens that adhere to deposits on the surface of the contact lens.

The Patient's Hands

The contact lens fitter should note the state of the patient's hands at the initial fitting visit, or indeed at the prefitting consultation. Long, sharp fingernails can not only damage the lenses but also cut the lids, conjunctiva, or cornea during lens insertion. Dirty fingers are vehicles of infection. Fungal lesions of the skin or nails indicate poor personal hygiene. Rheumatic changes of the fingers and hands may impede safe lens insertion and removal. Allergic changes on the skin imply that contact lens wearing may also be complicated by allergy.

The Lens Case

The lens case should be inspected at each follow-up visit. A dirty lens case implies that lens hygiene is probably deficient. Fingerprints on the lens case are, perhaps, tolerable, but actual dirt serves as an excellent reservoir for microbes that can then be transferred by the patient's finger into the eye during lens insertion. A leaky case cannot assure sterility; bubbles or crystalline deposits inside the case implies that the patient is too sparing with storage solution and changes it too infrequently to assure adequate disinfection of the lenses. Cloudiness, streaks, or even visible remnants of lens deposits inside the lens case clearly indicate that the patient is not treating the lenses with the necessary care.

Lens fragments or even several entire lenses swimming in the basin of the lens case indicate that the patient has been attempting to spare disinfecting solution.

Inspection of the lens case yields a clear indication of the adequacy of the patient's lens hygiene. Microbial cultures of the lens case are also advisable as an occasional screening test, and, of course, mandatory if any ocular complication should arise.

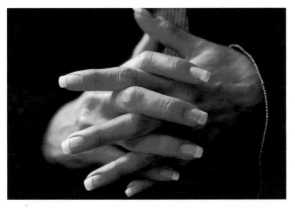

Fig. **298**   Sharp fingernails: a cause of corneal injury and resultant infection.

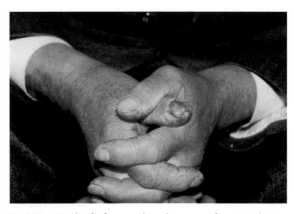

Fig. **299**   Hands of a farm worker who wore soft contact lenses and suffered from recurrent *Pseudomonas* infections of the eyes.

300

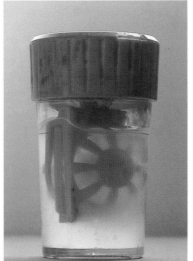

301

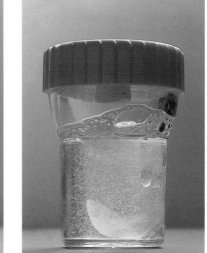

302

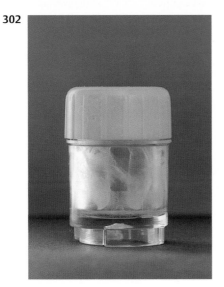

303

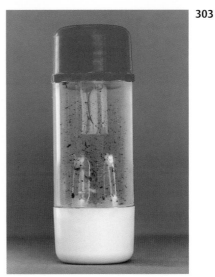

Fig. **300**   The lens case of a patient with a corneal ulcer. Note the proteinaceous debris in the storage fluid.

Fig. **301**   Very dirty lens from a patient with a corneal ulcer; positive culture for *Pseudomonas*.

Fig. **302**   Very dirty lens case of a patient with chronic conjunctivitis.

Fig. **303**   Soiled lens case of a construction worker; positive cultures for *Pseudomonas* and *Staphylococcus* from the surface and *Aspergillus niger* from the interior.

Wearing Times

The time a contact lens can safely remain on the eye is limited, as is the life of the lens itself.

If a lens is kept on the eye for too long without interruption, it can cause corneal epithelial edema and an increase in pachymetric values, while the patient complains of increased glare (an important warning sign). Such findings imply that the metabolic tolerance of contact lens wear has been exceeded, and that the continued presence of the lens on the eye will be dangerous.

Similar considerations apply to lenses worn past their useful life. Deposition of foreign matter in the interior of the lens and on its surface markedly decreases the oxygen permeability (Dk) of old lenses, leading in turn to diminished comfort and more frequent complications. The fitter must be aware of such problems and communicate them to the patient.

It is particularly important not to exceed the recommended wearing time when contact lenses are worn for medical indications, for example recurrent corneal erosion or bullous keratopathy, which are treated with contact lenses that remain on the eye without interruption for days or even months. Overwear syndrome and tight lens syndrome are among the more common reasons why such treatments may be prematurely discontinued. Regular follow-up at short intervals and frequent changing of the lenses help prevent these problems.

Fitting Errors

Poorly fitted lenses cause both mechanical and metabolic damage to the cornea, the latter because of impaired tear fluid convection and the resulting oxygen deficiency. Lens fitting must take the dynamic properties of the lens into account: the lens must be able to glide freely over the cornea during blinking, eye closure, and saccades. As shown in Illustration **9**, a steeply fitted hard lens can produce a circular impression on the epithelium and a central corneal deformation. Flatly fitted lenses cause central corneal flattening and corneal thinning and may produce corneal distortion syndrome (see pp. 125, 126). Very flatly fitted lens can probably also cause various forms of keratoconus. Unproblematic long-term contact lens wear can only be assured by meticulous fitting and regular follow-up examination with the ophthalmometer or keratometer, or with computerized topography.

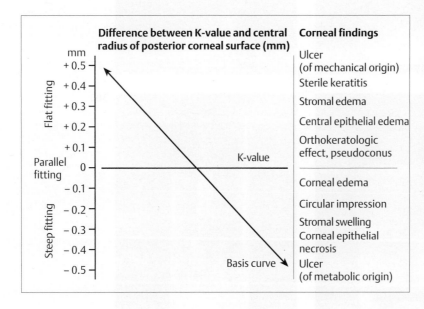

Illustration 9   Types of corneal injury caused by faulty fitting of rigid contact lenses. The more the radius of curvature of the posterior surface of the contact lens differs from that of the anterior surface of the cornea (K-value), the greater the resulting corneal deformation. Flat fitting causes central flattening and thinning of the cornea, possibly leading to pseudokeratoconus; steep fitting causes central corneal hypoxia, possibly leading to tissue defects. Either type of faulty fitting can lead, in extreme cases, to destruction of the optical center of the cornea, and to corneal infection.

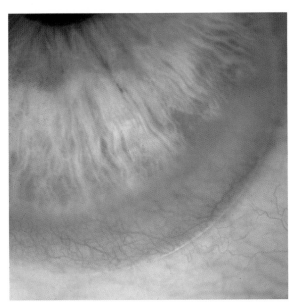

Fig. **304** Soft contact lens fitted too steeply; compression of the limbal sulcus.

305

306

307

308

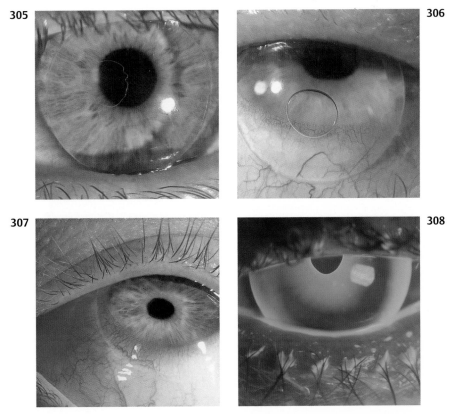

Fig. **305** High-Dk rigid gas-permeable (RGP) lens fitted too steeply; paracentral air bubble in the tear lens.

Fig. **307** Soft hydrophilic lens fitted too steeply and compressing the perilimbal conjunctiva.

Fig. **306** Hard CAB lens fitted too steeply and caudally displaced; large air bubble under the lens.

Fig. **308** Soft silicone lens fitted too steeply; pooling of fluorescein under the central part of the lens; bubble in the tear lens.

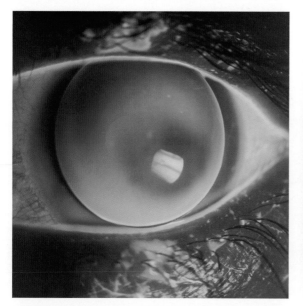

Fig. **309** CAB lens for keratoconus, fitted too flatly; paracentral fluorescein-free area.

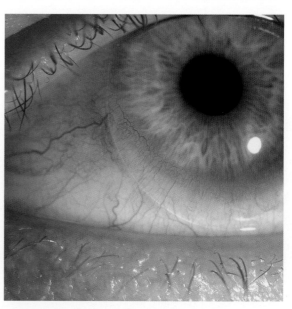

Fig. **310** Soft PMMA lens in stage 2 keratoconus in unacceptable, decentered position (inferiorly displaced).

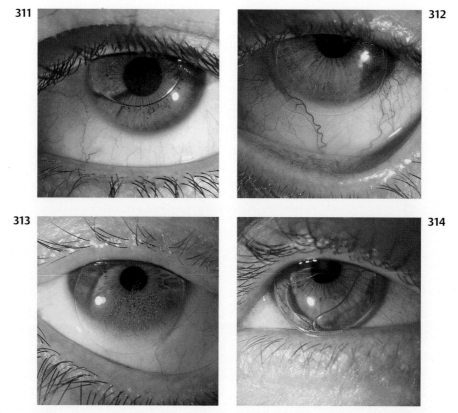

Fig. **311** Hard contact lens for keratoconus, fitted too flatly; paracentral pressure area.

Fig. **312** Soft silicone lens fitted too flatly and inferiorly displaced; conjunctival injection.

Fig. **313** Hard lens for myopia; inferiorly displaced; fitted too steeply; air bubbles in the tear lens.

Fig. **314** Hard lens for keratoconus fit extremely flatly; ring-like air bubble under the lens periphery.

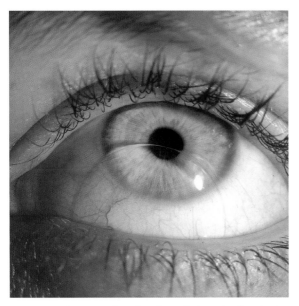 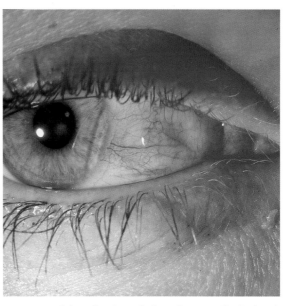

Fig. **315** Soft contact lens fitted too flatly and inferiorly displaced; excessive mobility on blinking.

Fig. **316** Soft lens fitted too flatly and temporally displaced; focal irritation of the conjunctiva.

6 Alterations of Contact Lenses

Wetting Problems

Material Defects

Discoloration and Fading

Deposits

Components of the Tear Fluid

Jelly Bumps

Wetting Problems

Symptoms: Fluctuations in visual acuity associated with blinking.

Clinical findings: Inadequate wetting of the lens surface; abnormal break-up time (BUT) on the lens surface.

Transient visual impairment associated with blinking implies a disturbance of wetting of the eye or of the contact lens surface. Glare is produced by cloudiness of the lens surface, the interior of the lens, or the refractive media of the eye.

Visual impairment lasting 10–20 minutes after lens insertion in the morning may also indicate a wetting problem, as tear flow is normally less during sleep. Such problems can be dealt with by instillation of artificial tears upon awakening, before the physiological inflow of tears starts. Wetting the lens after insertion may also solve the problem. Impaired vision during the day accompanied by cloudiness or glare may be a sign of early corneal edema or giant papillary conjunctivitis (GPC); these conditions are readily diagnosed with the slit lamp.

Visual impairment can result from disorders of lacrimation and the dry-eye syndrome. Any abnormality of the quality or quantity of tear fluid can impair vision in a contact lens wearer. Soft lenses need a reservoir of tears to retain their elasticity; hard lenses need a cushion of tears so that they can glide freely over the corneal surface. The tear lens between the contact lens and the cornea can only form if adequate tear fluid is present; the tear lens is an optical medium in itself and, depending on its geometry, serves as an additional plano, convex, or concave lens that cancels out small astigmatic errors. Thus, any change in the refractive index of the tear fluid, caused by fluctuations of its osmolarity, pH, or salt content, may affect visual function (cf. p. 128).

Material Defects

A contact lens can be worn safely and comfortably only if its surface is smooth, that is, free of nicks, scratches, tears, sharp-edged defects, fracture lines, deposits, or foreign bodies. All of these abnormalities can cause an uncomfortable foreign-body sensation.

Surface deposits serve as a culture medium for microbial pathogens and thereby promote infection. They also impair the wettability of the lens surface, which leads, in turn, to impaired vision and increased glare. Surface deposits must be removed from the lenses before each insertion, and defective lenses must be discarded. Patients wearing disposable lenses, in particular, should be reminded of these important facts at each follow-up visit, as these are precisely the patients that tend to wear their lenses much longer than recommended by the manufacturer.

Defective contact lenses can injure the lids, conjunctiva, and cornea. Hyperemia or hemorrhage of the tarsal or bulbar conjunctiva, and corneal epithelial defects, are usually caused by wearing contact lenses past their wearable lifetimes.

All contact lenses deteriorate over time and are therefore meant to be worn for a limited time only. Lens manufacturers do not guarantee their lenses for any specific length of time, but the general recommendation is that soft lenses should be worn for no longer than 1 year, hard lenses for no longer than 2 years. Contact lenses should be discarded at the end of their wearable lifetime and replaced with new ones. Disposable, one-day, and reusable lenses should be worn for no longer than 24 hours, a few days, and a few weeks, respectively. Patient compliance with these guidelines is, unfortunately, often suboptimal. Disposable lenses that have been worn too long are often broken, discolored, or deformed; fatigue fractures (stress lines) are seen in the lens matrix, the rim of the lens is broken or torn, and tenacious deposits are found on its surface. All of these findings indicate that the tolerance of the contact lens material for prolonged wear has been exceeded.

Fine scratches on the anterior surface of hard lenses are only rarely disturbing; these can arise simply from the lens being worn in the eye, but may also be caused by mechanical cleaning with bare fingers. If the lens is well wetted, these defects are optically compensated for by the tear fluid, and are thus barely noted at first. They are disturbing only if they exceed a certain size so that they irritate the cornea or impair vision. If this occurs, it is time to replace the lens.

Some types of highly gas-permeable rigid lenses are prone to the development of a mosaic pattern on their surface which resembles a smashed windshield. This change usually occurs after a relatively long period of wear; if it is found shortly after fitting, it is presumably due to a manufacturing error. Such patterns are probably created by too rapid cooling of the lens material in the polymerization process.

At each follow-up visit, the contact lenses should be inspected under a dissecting microscope, or under a slit lamp with the aid of an inverting prism. The inspection can be performed in white light, but the use of polarized light will facilitate early detection of stress lines and other defects. Surface and edge defects are very reliably detected by Zeiss dark field examination in cold light.

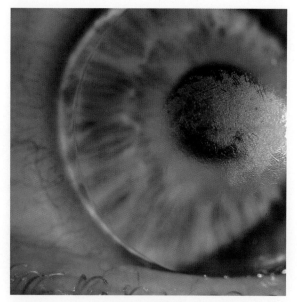

Fig. **317** Scratches on a hard CAB lens.

318

319

320

321

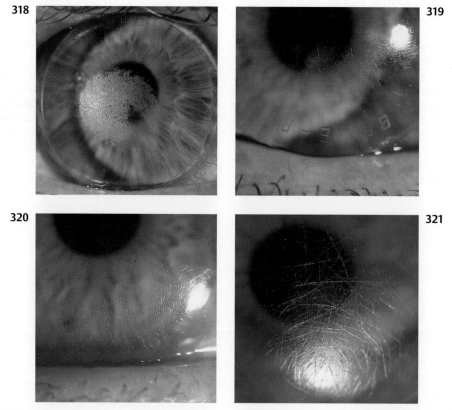

Fig. **318** Scratches on a hard fluorosilicone carbonate lens.

Fig. **319** Scratches on a hard PMMA lens.

Fig. **320** Fine superficial cracks on a hard contact lens; aging of the material.

Fig. **321** Scratches on a hard lens. Faulty cleaning and aging of the lens surface.

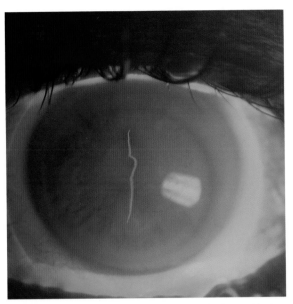

Fig. 322 Central fracture in a worn-out soft disposable lens (worn for 16 months). Fluorescein stain.

323

324

325

326

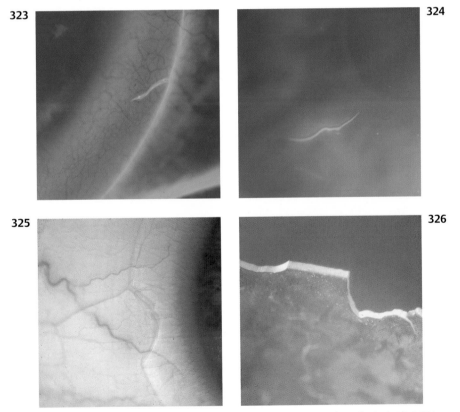

Fig. 323 Cracked edge of a 2-year-old soft contact lens.

Fig. 325 Sharp broken edge of a 4-year-old soft contact lens.

Fig. 324 Cracked edge of a high-Dk RGP lens, about 3 years old.

Fig. 326 Edge defect in a soft contact lens; slit-lamp image, X30.

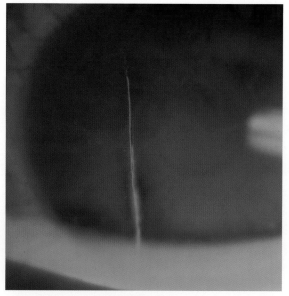

Fig. **327** Horizontal tear in a soft lens of high water content, due to improper handling. Fluorescein stain.

328

329

330

331

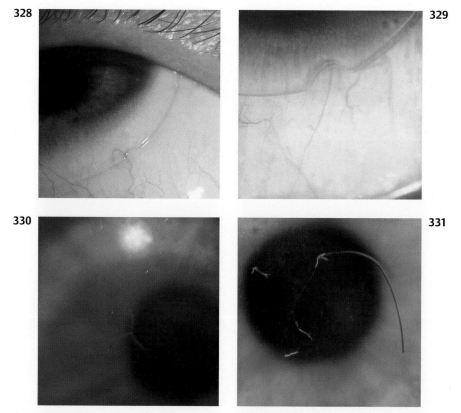

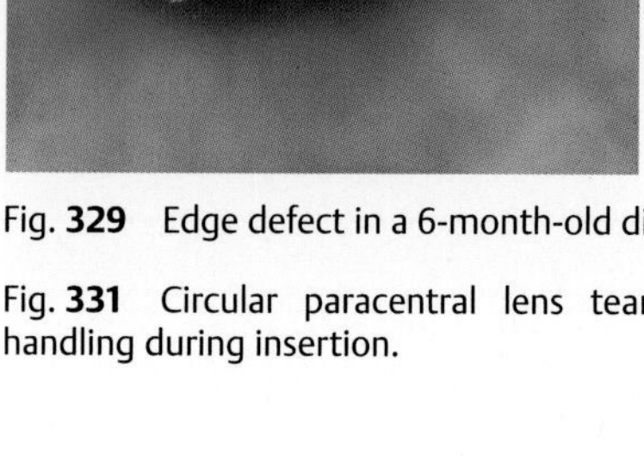

Fig. **328** Flawed edge of a soft lens of high water content, about 3 years old.

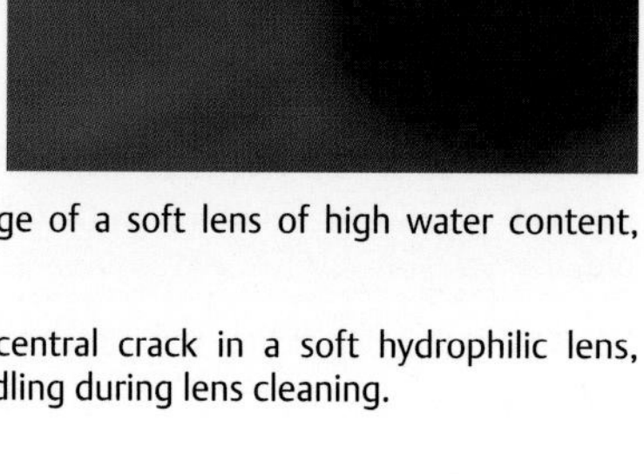

Fig. **330** Y-shaped central crack in a soft hydrophilic lens, caused by faulty handling during lens cleaning.

Fig. **329** Edge defect in a 6-month-old disposable lens.

Fig. **331** Circular paracentral lens tear, caused by faulty handling during insertion.

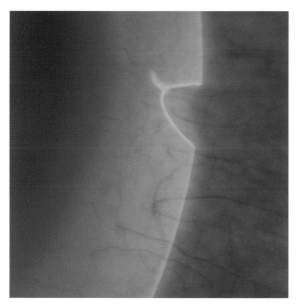

Fig. **332** Single-use soft contact lens; fluorescein staining; edge defect caused by faulty handling during insertion.

333

334

335

336

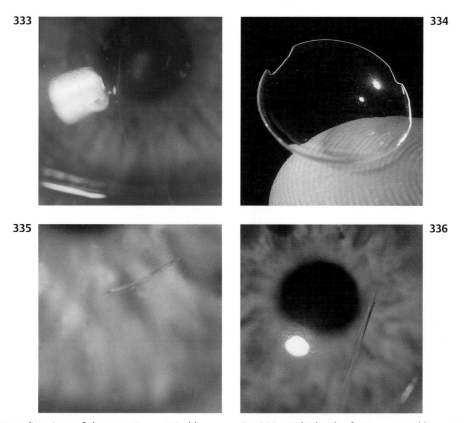

Fig. **333** Fracture lines in a soft lens creating a stainable corneal epithelial defect.

Fig. **335** Central fissures in a soft hydrophilic contact lens, caused by drying out and rehydration.

Fig. **334** Multiple edge fractures resembling a circular saw in a soft 1-month lens worn for 14 months.

Fig. **336** Fatigue fracture in a soft 1-month lens that was worn for 32 months.

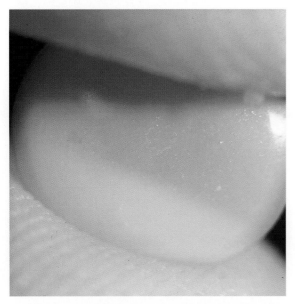

Fig. **337** Total opacification of a hard lens made of fluorosilicone carbonate, cause unknown.

338

339

340

341

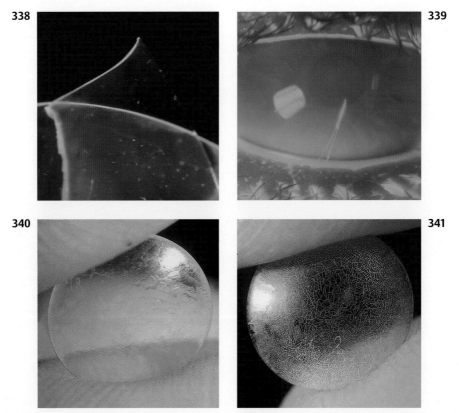

Fig. **338** Soft, disposable lens that broke after 1 hour of wear; manufacturing error.

Fig. **340** Deposits on the surface of a hard lens, which has become hydrophobic; manufacturing error.

Fig. **339** Paracentral fissure in a rigid lens due to faulty handling.

Fig. **341** Cracks in a high-Dk RGP lens due to an error in tempering.

Discoloration and Fading

Most contact lenses become discolored with wear because of a change in the molecular structure of the lens material over time. In general, soft hydrophilic lenses turn yellowish-brown after they have been worn for a number of years. The discoloration is harmless in itself but serves as a marker for an accompanying decline in gas permeability. Thus, discolored lenses should be replaced.

Eye make-up in all colors is often found on the anterior surface of contact lenses and is not always removable. Lenses rinsed with tap water of high iron content develop a brown hue. The soft lenses of cigarette smokers are often stained reddish-brown to an extent that reflects how much they have smoked; those of firemen turn rust-brown after repeated exposure to the chemical substances liberated in fires (see Table **26**). Lenses that have become discolored by external substances in this manner should be replaced, as the risk of toxic keratopathy from re-release of the adsorbed substances is difficult to assess. Patients at risk for such problems (heavy smokers, firemen, others) should wear disposable lenses.

Oral, parenteral, or even topical medications can discolor soft contact lenses, particularly when they are used to treat ophthalmic diseases, such as recurrent corneal erosions or bullous keratopathy.

Many different types of dyed and painted lenses are now commercially available; they are used to occlude the eye, to mask ocular birth defects or traumatic lesions, to reduce glare in aniridia or fixed mydriasis, or for elective cosmetic purposes. The last few years have witnessed the rising popularity of so-called party lenses with surface designs such as cat's eyes, hearts, flowers, and dollar signs. The coloring of such lenses is not necessarily stable and may leach out of the lens to cause an allergic or toxic reaction.

Table **26** Causes of lens staining

Color of staining	Causes
White, bright gray	Proteins, lipids, mucopolysaccharides, calcium, jelly bumps, fungi, medications
Dark gray, black	Thiomersal, mercuric compounds
Red	Iron, fungi, tap water, medications
Pink	Vitamin B12, antibiotics
Yellow	Cosmetics, aging of lens material
Brown	Nicotine, fumes from fires, cosmetics, sprays
Green	Sorbic acid (a preservative), algae, chlorhexidine
Blue	Cosmetics

Tinted, light-absorbing lenses are medically indicated in certain forms of retinal degeneration, and in albinism. They can also be worn for cosmetic purposes to change the color of the eye to blue, green, or brown according to the whim of the wearer. These lenses slowly fade over time; fading may be accelerated by the use of inappropriate lens care products, such as hydrogen peroxide, which acts as a bleach.

It is not known with certainty whether the chemical dyes used could, in some circumstances, pose a risk to the cornea and conjunctiva. These substances should be remembered in the differential diagnosis of allergic and toxic reactions in the contact lens wearer; the Ophthalmotest may help resolve the issue (see p. 80).

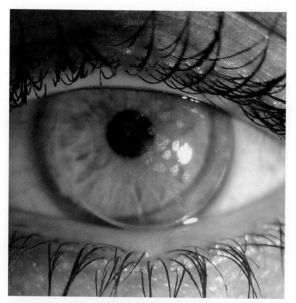

Fig. **342**   Make-up residue on the surface of a hard lens. A typical instance of faulty cleaning.

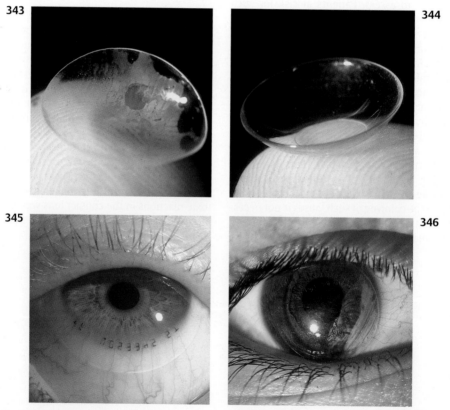

Fig. **343**   Cloudy areas of a soft contact lens cleaned with an unknown household cleaner. Improper lens care.

Fig. **345**   Coloring of the engraving on a soft contact lens by eyeliner pigment.

Fig. **344**   Rust-brown staining of a CAB lens worn during a major fire in a chemical laboratory (responsible substance unknown).

Fig. **346**   Destruction of the surface of a hard lens by nail polish remover (contains acetone).

Deposits

Substances from the environment are deposited on the anterior surface of the contact lens. Solids, including foreign bodies, remain there, while liquids penetrate into the lens itself, and gases are dissolved in the tear film and transported by it around and into the lens. Only meticulous daily cleaning and disinfection can prevent long-term damage from such substances.

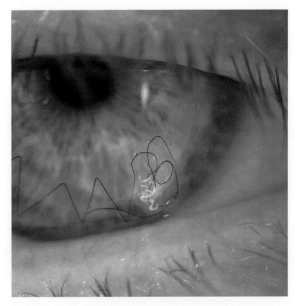

Fig. 347 Broken suture after corneal graft. Wearing a soft contact lens; marked foreign body irritation.

348

349

350

351

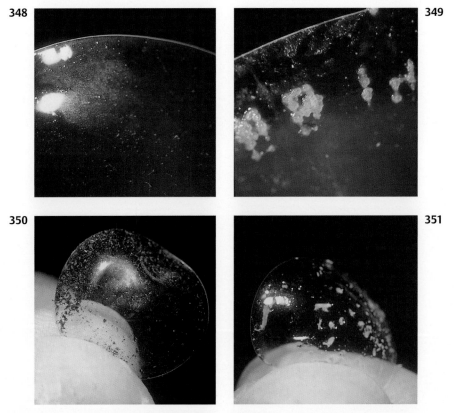

Fig. 348 Deposits on the irregular surface of a soft contact lens; dark-field image.

Fig. 349 Jelly-bump-like residue of clear varnish in the engraving of a contact lens; dark-field image.

Fig. 350 Metallic dust on a soft lens worn in the workplace without protective goggles.

Fig. 351 Sawdust on a soft contact lens worn in a carpenter's shop.

352

353

354

355

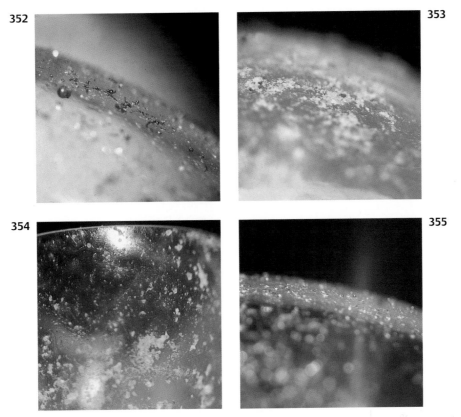

Fig. **352** Deposits of molten metal on a hard contact lens worn by a welder without protective goggles.

Fig. **354** Hairspray residue on the surface of a soft lens.

Fig. **353** Flour on a soft contact lens worn in a bakery.

Fig. **355** Metallic particles on the surface of a soft lens.

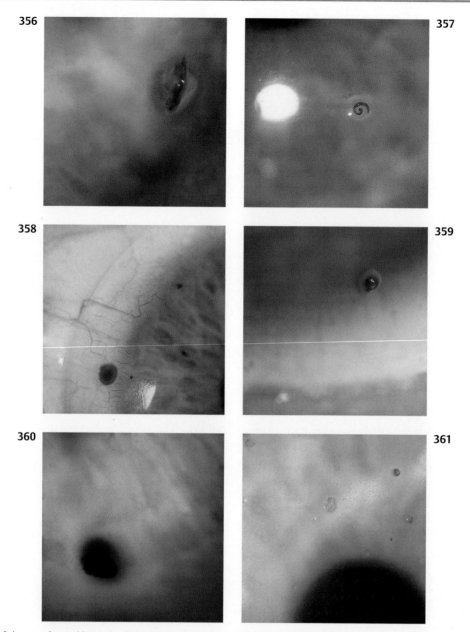

Fig. **356**   Soft lens perforated by a metallic splinter.

Fig. **358**   Rusted metallic foreign body at the edge of a soft contact lens.

Fig. **360**   Rusted metallic foreign body in a soft contact lens.

Fig. **357**   Iron spring embedded in the surface of a soft contact lens.

Fig. **359**   Rusted metallic foreign body in a soft contact lens.

Fig. **361**   Multiple rust-like deposits on a soft contact lens *(Aspergillus niger).*

Components of Tear Fluid

Not only environmental pollutants, but also components of the tear fluid leave their mark on the lens, as seen under the slit lamp. The tear fluid normally contains proteins, lipids, and desquamated cellular debris from the cornea and conjunctiva, all of which are deposited on the surface of the contact lens during the daily period of wear. If these deposits are allowed to accumulate, they can impair vision, increase glare, and mechanically irritate the eyelids, making lens wear uncomfortable (see p. 66). They can also decrease lens wettability and cause GPC.

These organic deposits can also promote infection; kept moist by the tear fluid and the matrix of hydrophilic lenses, they serve as a bacterial and fungal culture medium. Dirty lenses confer a particularly high risk of infection.

A special form of contact lens deposit has been termed the "sock phenomenon." Proteinaceous deposits on the posterior surface of the lens can decrease its mobility by, in essence, gluing it to the cornea. The name is derived from the appearance of the deposits along the lens edges under the slit lamp (they are said to resemble socks on a clothesline). This phenomenon is rare, and its cause is unknown.

Jelly Bumps

Jelly bumps are small grayish-white deposits that appear to be spattered on the anterior surface of the lens. Microscopic or slit-lamp examination reveals their crystalline or onion-skin structure. They are hardly ever seen on the inner surface of the lens. They may appear singly or dispersed over the surface of the lens like stars in the night sky.

Jelly bumps are commonly found on soft lenses, rarely on hard lenses. The water content and chemical structure of the lens material determine whether they will form. The more hydrophilic the lens, the more rapidly jelly bumps are deposited; deposition is also promoted by poor-quality material and by defects of the lens surface such as scratches, grooves, and polishing flaws. Jelly bumps make blinking uncomfortable because they irritate the lid margin. They are hard to remove and they recur rapidly if they are due to a structural defect of the lens. Such lenses should be replaced.

Jelly bumps are composed of water-insoluble calcium–protein complexes. This explains both how they are generated and why they are so difficult to remove. In addition to the defective contact lens, the concentration of calcium in the tear fluid is another important determinant of their formation.

Pregnant and breastfeeding women and those taking oral contraceptives develop jelly bumps more rapidly than others; so do patients with parathyroid disorders or hypercalcemia of other causes, as well as patients being treated with medications affecting calcium metabolism or high-dose hormones or oral antibiotics. In some cases, new jelly bumps can be seen as early as a few hours after lens insertion.

There remains no effective way to prevent the formation of jelly bumps. Intensive cleaning, sometimes with highly concentrated cleaning solutions, is frequently recommended, but should in fact be avoided, because residues of the cleaning chemicals may be stored in hydrophilic lenses and may then interact with the patient's lens care solution.

Patients prone to the development of jelly bumps should avoid wearing highly hydrophilic lenses to minimize the risk of such problems. A switch to rigid gas-permeable (RGP) lenses or soft lenses with less than 40% content usually renders the patient asymptomatic. Because of the association between jelly bumps and disorders of calcium metabolism, patients with recurrent jelly bumps should have their serum calcium level determined. Any abnormality should be followed up with a general medical evaluation.

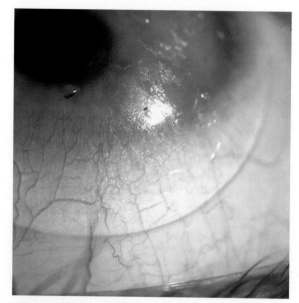

Fig. **362** Dense proteinaceous deposits on a soft lens; poor lens hygiene.

363

364

365

366

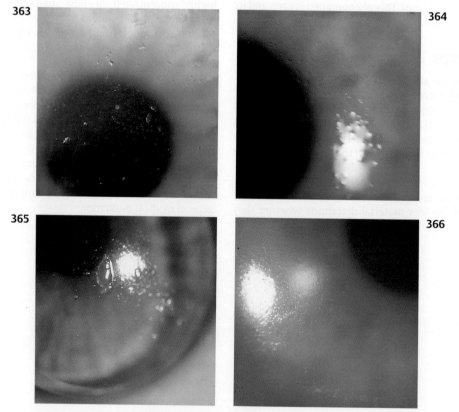

Fig. **363** Proteinaceous deposits on the surface of a worn-out hard CAB lens.

Fig. **364** Lipid deposits on the anterior surface of a worn-out fluorosilicone carbonate lens.

Fig. **365** Droplets of fat and protein on a hard contact lens; poor lens hygiene.

Fig. **366** Protein coating on a soft contact lens; poor lens hygiene.

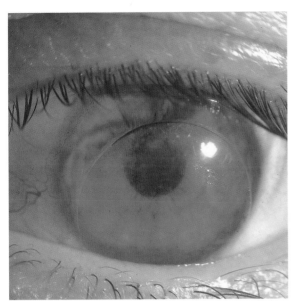

Fig. **367** CAB lens densely coated with protein in an allergic patient during the hay-fever season. Risk of GPC.

368

369

370

371

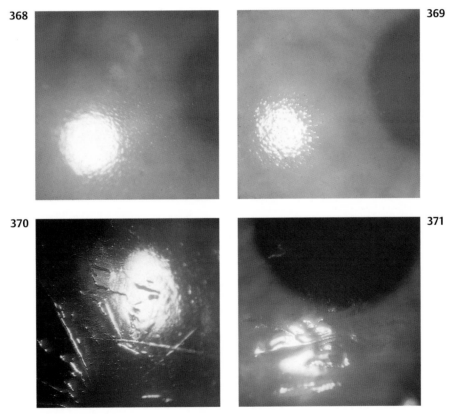

Fig. **368** Dense proteinaceous deposits on a 4-year-old soft contact lens.

Fig. **369** Dense proteinaceous deposits on a 6-year-old soft contact lens.

Fig. **370** Dense proteinaceous deposits on a soft contact lens; hydrophobic surface. Aging of the lens material.

Fig. **371** Dense proteinaceous deposits on a soft contact lens; hydrophobic surface. Aging of the lens material, faulty cleaning.

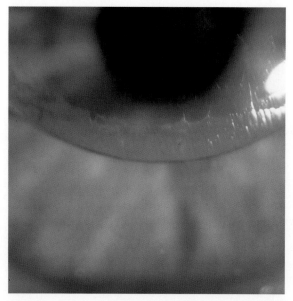

Fig. **372** Sock phenomenon; lens stuck to the cornea because of abnormal proteinaceous deposits.

373

374

375

376

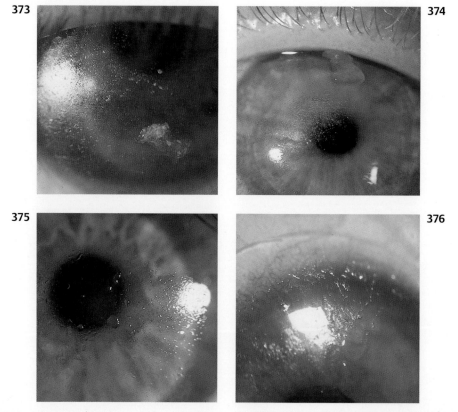

Fig. **373** Dense proteinaceous deposits on a soft contact lens; faulty cleaning.

Fig. **375** Proteinaceous deposits on a soft contact lens; faulty cleaning.

Fig. **374** Dense, sock-like proteinaceous deposits on the surface of a soft lens; sock phenomenon.

Fig. **376** Proteinaceous deposits on a hard contact lens; poor lens care.

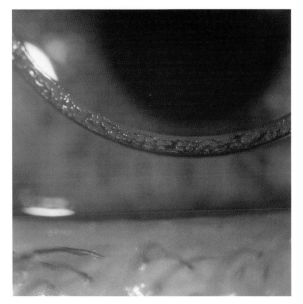

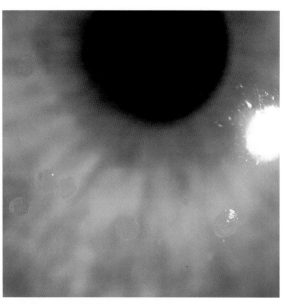

Fig. **377** Proteinaceous deposits on the edge of an RGP lens, causing foreign body sensation.

Fig. **378** Jelly bumps on a soft contact lens; surface damage; faulty cleaning.

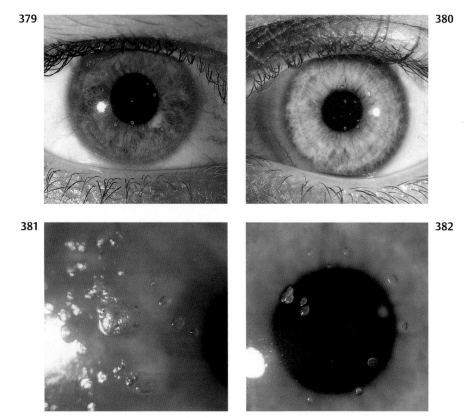

Fig. **379** Jelly bumps on a soft contact lens; faulty cleaning.

Fig. **380** Jelly bumps on a soft contact lens; poor hygiene.

Fig. **381** Jelly bumps on a soft contact lens; disorder of calcium metabolism.

Fig. **382** Jelly bumps on a soft contact lens; developed after only a few days of hormone therapy.

383

384

385

386

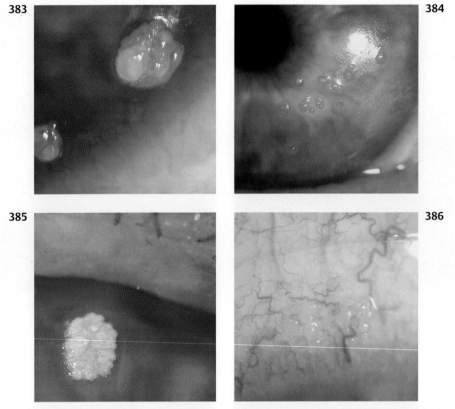

Fig. **383** Jelly bumps on a soft contact lens; material defect.

Fig. **385** Isolated jelly bump deposited on the defective surface of a soft contact lens.

Fig. **384** Jelly bumps on a soft lens of high water content; defective material.

Fig. **386** Jelly bumps in the engraving of a soft hydrophilic contact lens.

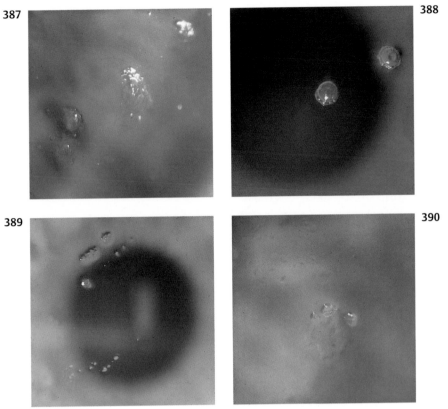

Fig. **387**   Jelly bumps on a soft contact lens; tear deficiency; worn-out lens.

Fig. **388**   Jelly bumps on a soft disposable lens; tear deficiency; oral calcium supplementation; lens worn for 6 months.

Fig. **389**   Jelly bumps on a worn-out soft lens.

Fig. **390**   Jelly bumps on the defective surface of a worn-out soft lens.

7 Primary Fitting and Wearing Problems

Systemic Disease

Febrile Illnesses, Immune Compromise, Medication Use

Allergy

Primary Ocular Disease

Lid Diseases

Conjunctival Diseases

Corneal Diseases

Tear Deficiency, Disorders of Lacrimation, Dry Eye

Other Eye Diseases

Systemic Disease

Many systemic illnesses first manifest themselves in the eye or affect the eye secondarily. Many orally and parenterally administered medications gain access to the eye through the tear fluid and can adhere to the contact lens surface, accumulate in the hydrophilic stroma of soft lenses, and interact with the polymers of which the lenses are composed.

Febrile Illnesses, Immune Compromise, Medication Use

Fever elevates not only the core temperature, but also the temperature of the anterior ocular segment. Two consequences of this are a need for an increased amount of tear fluid and an alteration of the conjunctival flora. The normal temperature in the cul-de-sac is 35.6 $\pm$ 0.2 °C; a rise of as little as 1–2 °C creates a favorable environment for the growth of *Pseudomonas*, which explains why contact lens wearers are much more likely to develop *Pseudomonas* conjunctivitis or keratitis when suffering from a febrile illness, such as the common cold. Respiratory diseases such as bronchitis or bronchial pneumonia raise the incidence of acanthamoebal, fungal, and pneumococcal corneal ulcers in contact lens wearers.

Immune compromise of various causes, including AIDS, leukemia, and antineoplastic chemotherapy, predisposes to ocular infection. It is thus critical that contact lenses are not worn in such situations. Contact-lens-related complications are also more frequent in the presence of systemic diseases affecting the quality and quantity of tears, including thyroid, parathyroid, and other metabolic disorders and renal failure. Florid hepatitis may necessitate discontinuation of contact lenses, as may pregnancy or nursing, in rare cases.

Many orally or parenterally administered medications enter the tear fluid and affect wearing comfort. Beta-blockers and hormones are the most prominent examples. The effects of oral contraceptives have already been discussed (p. 5). Coagulopathies or therapeutic anticoagulation can result in massive conjunctival hemorrhage during lens insertion or removal, or indeed while the lenses are worn, after minor trauma to blood vessels of the anterior segment.

In patients with active or even latent diabetes mellitus, there is a significantly more frequent colonization of the cornea and conjunctiva with fungi such as *Candida* and *Aspergillus*, and a correspondingly higher frequency of fungal infection.

Allergy

Any allergic predisposition may complicate the wearing of contact lenses. Patients who are allergic to synthetic materials in general usually cannot tolerate any type of contact lens material. Patients with ectopic dermatitis may rapidly develop blepharitis after contact lenses are inserted, while patients with allergic vasomotor rhinitis may develop allergic blepharoconjunctivitis or keratopathy. Those who suffer from hay fever can rarely wear their lenses comfortably at the critical times of year.

Primary Ocular Disease

Many ocular diseases can complicate the wearing of contact lenses. The contact lenses themselves, as well as lens care products and wetting solutions, may evoke an allergic response. Ocular infections can become more severe in the presence of contact lenses or be spread by the contact lenses to critical areas of the cornea. It is unknown at present whether premalignant ocular lesions are more likely to transform into malignancy when contact lenses are worn, but unnecessary risks should not be taken; thus, any pigmented spots on the lids or conjunctiva should be noted and photographically documented before fitting, and followed up at regular intervals thereafter.

Tear deficiency causes innumerable complications in contact lens wearers; if severe, tear deficiency absolutely contraindicates contact lens wear. The diagnosis and treatment of dry eye is not always a simple matter. The most important acute and chronic ocular diseases that may affect contact lens wear are listed in Tables **27** and **28**.

Lid Diseases

Acute infections of the lids, conjunctiva, and cornea complicate contact lens wear. Hordeolum and (more rarely) lid abscess necessitate temporary discontinuation of contact lenses, as the lenses might otherwise be a vector for the spread of pathogenic bacteria to the cornea.

Chalazion, in its early infectious phase, poses the same risk to the contact wearer as hordeolum and necessitates temporary discontinuation of contact lenses. In its inactive phase, after healing and encapsulation, it may still be a mechanical hindrance to contact lens wear.

Chronic blepharitis is a major problem. Of the many etiological forms of chronic blepharitis, allergic squamous blepharitis is the most likely to develop in contact lens wearers because of an allergy to the lenses or to lens care products. Regardless of treatment, such patients hardly ever tolerate their lenses well over the long term.

Chronic, recurrent lid edema of any cause interferes with the lie of the lens on the eye. Contact lens wearers with this problem complain of a foreign body sensation and generally cannot wear contact lenses over the long term.

The lie of the lens is also disturbed by ectropion or entropion, as well as by post-traumatic or postsurgical alterations of lid function. Scarring of the lid margin after trauma or infection, lid paresis, or malposition of the punctum can interfere with the flow of tears and thereby

Table 27 Acute ocular diseases interfering with contact lens wear

Lid trauma
New or infected piercing
Purulent blepharitis
Lid herpes
Hordeolum
Stye
Bacterial, fungal, and viral conjunctivitis
Conjunctival trauma
Corneal trauma
Toxic keratopathy
Bacterial, fungal, or viral keratitis
Intraocular infection
Acute glaucoma
Previous eye surgery

Table 28 Chronic ocular diseases interfering with contact lens wear

Lid scarring
Malposition of the lids
Defects of the lid margin
Extensive pinguecula
Chalazion
Chronic recurrent hordeola
Chronic conjunctivitis
Conjunctival malformations or neoplasia
Filter blebs
Recurrent keratitis or uveitis

complicate contact lens wear. Patients with these problems usually have to stop wearing contact lenses soon after the initial fitting because of a pronounced foreign body sensation and frequent lens loss.

Eyelashes that point inward scrape the cornea and conjunctiva with each lid movement, irritating the anterior ocular segment. If a contact lens is worn, they push it back and forth over the cornea. This condition must be excluded or, if present, corrected before contact lenses are fitted.

Lid function and the lie of the contact lens can be adversely affected by any malignant or benign mass of the eyelid, such as a papilloma or sebaceous cyst. Before contact lenses are fitted, such masses should be excised.

391

392

393

394

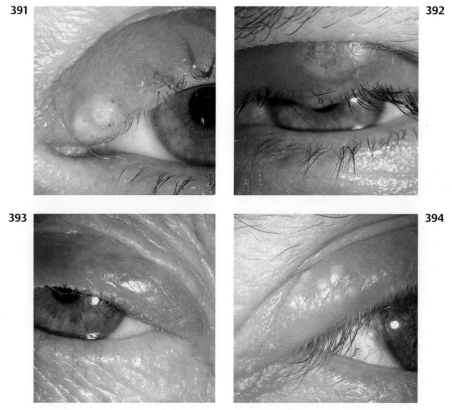

Fig. **391** Hordeolum, upper lid.

Fig. **393** Herpes, upper lid margin.

Fig. **392** Ulcerated chalazion on the upper lid, infectious process.

Fig. **394** Herpes simplex, upper lid.

395

396

397

398

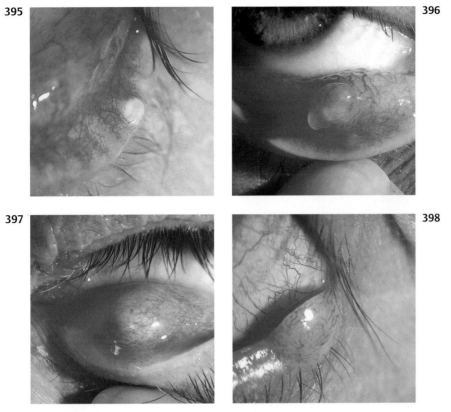

Fig. **395** Conjunctival cyst, tarsal conjunctiva of lower lid.

Fig. **396** Cyst, inner surface of lower lid.

Fig. **397** Internal chalazion, lower lid.

Fig. **398** Benign tumor of the lower lid margin.

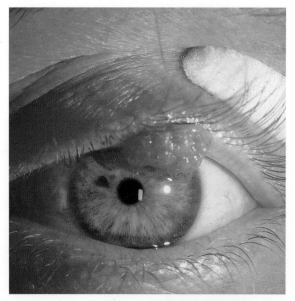

Fig. **399** Lid margin papilloma, center of upper lid.

400

401

402

403

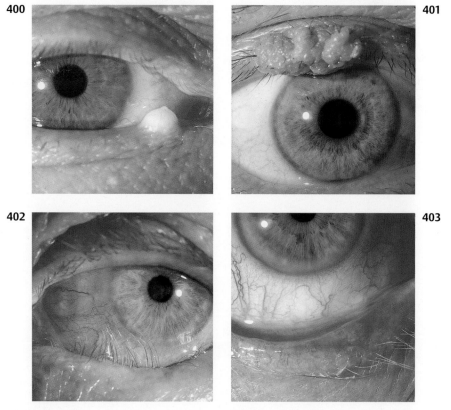

Fig. **400** Milium, inner canthus, lower lid.

Fig. **401** Wart, central upper lid margin.

Fig. **402** Entropion, lower lid.

Fig. **403** Ectropion, lower lid.

Conjunctival Diseases

Acute or chronic conjunctivitis of any etiology absolutely contraindicates contact lens wear. Wearing contact lenses in this situation would not only create an intense foreign body sensation but would also be likely to exacerbate the disease process by provoking additional inflammation. Innumerable cases of corneal ulceration in contact lens wearers have occurred on the background of prior bacterial, fungal, or viral conjunctivitis. Conjunctival cuts, hemorrhages, edema, or lesions should be allowed to heal completely before lens wear is resumed.

Conjunctival growths, such as pingueculae or pigmented spots, often cause mechanical problems. It remains an unresolved question whether the mechanical irritation caused by a contact lens can promote the transformation of a pigmented spot to a malignant process (melanoma). It would seem prudent to remove any nevus that might be touched by a contact lens before the lens is fitted.

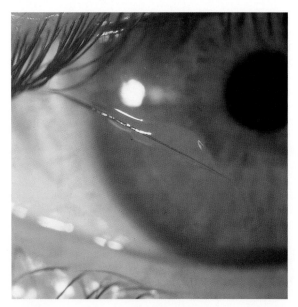

Fig. **404** Distichiasis, lash abrading the cornea, foreign body sensation.

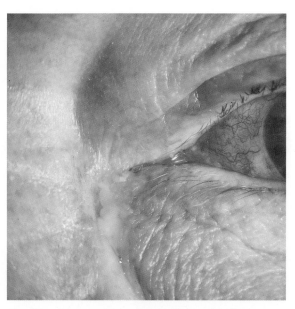

Fig. **405** Dacryocystitis, occlusion of lacrimal pathway.

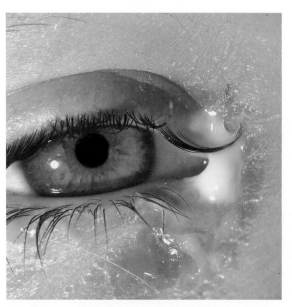

Fig. **406** Dacryocystitis, occlusion of lacrimal pathway.

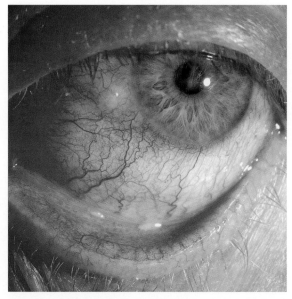

Fig. **407** Chronic bacterial conjunctivitis.

408

409

410

411

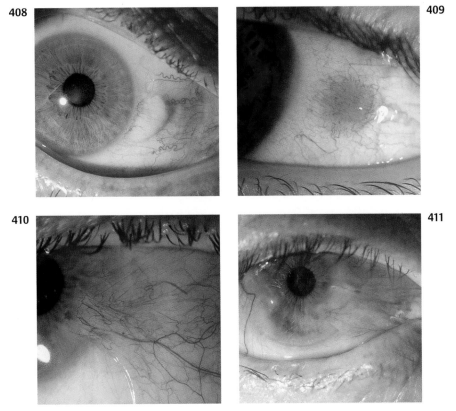

Fig. **408** Pinguecula, conjunctival erosion from the edge of a hard contact lens, stained with rose bengal.

Fig. **410** Pseudopterygium from keratitis.

Fig. **409** Conjunctival phlyctena.

Fig. **411** Pseudopterygium from alkali burn.

412

413

414

415

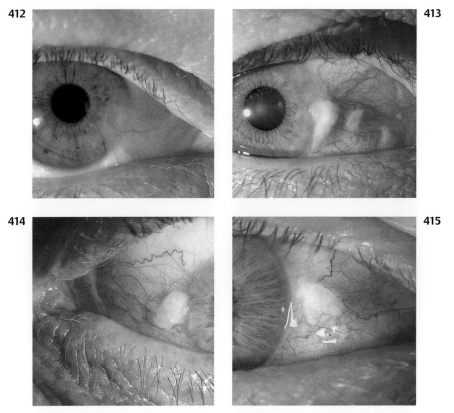

Fig. **412** Pterygium.

Fig. **413** Conjunctival papilloma adjacent to the limbus.

Fig. **414** Conjunctival tumor adjacent to the limbus.

Fig. **415** Conjunctival tumor adjacent to the limbus.

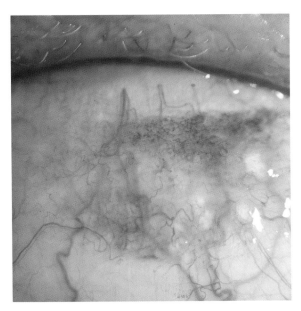

Fig. **416** Conjnctival nevus, benign.

417

418

419

420

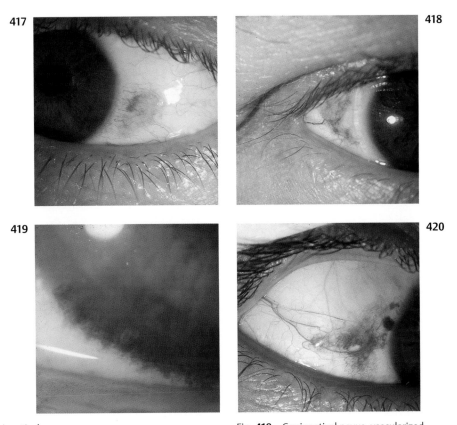

Fig. **417** Conjunctival nevus.

Fig. **418** Conjunctival nevus, vascularized.

Fig. **419** Conjunctival melanosis.

Fig. **420** Conjunctival melanoma.

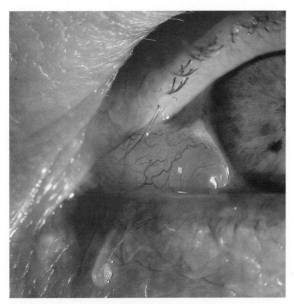

Fig. **421** Conjunctival cyst after a perforation of the bulb, aphakia.

422

423

424

425

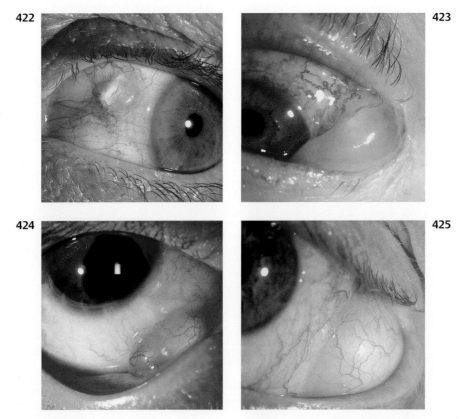

Fig. **422** Conjunctival cyst.

Fig. **424** Conjunctival cyst after perforation of the bulb.

Fig. **423** Conjunctival cyst with extension to the retrobulbar space.

Fig. **425** Prolapsed conjunctival fatty tissue.

Corneal Diseases

Corneal infections and acute corneal processes of any other type contraindicate the wearing of contact lenses. All contact lenses impair the metabolism of the cornea to some extent; though the disturbance is well tolerated by a healthy eye when modern lens systems are used, it is likely to contribute to the progression of any corneal disease that may be present. Within a few hours of being covered by a contact lens, keratitis can develop into a corneal ulcer, and corneal herpes can develop into metaherpetic keratitis.

The situation is somewhat different in deformities or degenerative diseases of the cornea, which are often, in fact, a medical indication for contact lenses. They may, however, give rise to major fitting problems, for example in the case of irregular astigmatism or keratoconus. If adequate centration and stabilization of the contact lens cannot be achieved, corrective corneal surgery may be required.

Recurrent corneal erosions contraindicate contact lens wear for cosmetic or optical indications, as contact lenses—particularly hard lenses—can repeatedly shear the poorly anchored epithelium from the underlying tissue, causing severe pain. Nonetheless, soft, ultra-thin bandage lenses are an excellent form of treatment for chronic recurrent erosions, as well as for bullous keratopathy, which is often accompanied by endothelial dystrophy. In summary, patients with these conditions should only wear contact lenses for therapeutic indications.

Tear Deficiency, Disorders of Lacrimation, Dry Eye

Symptoms: Feeling of dryness and grittiness; eye-rubbing; increased ocular temperature; glare.

Clinical findings: Persistent conjunctival injection; blurred vision; irregular changes of refractive error while lenses are worn.

Pathophysiology

The tear film serves multiple essential functions for normal vision, as listed in Table **29**. Most important is the delivery of nutrients to the avascular cornea and the preservation of physiological and biochemical homeostasis. As shown by recent basic research, the problems associated with tear deficiency that limit lens wear result primarily from nutrient deficiency of the cornea and conjunctiva.

Table **29**   Actions of the tear fluid
Protection against drying
Heat exchange, temperature regulation
Transport of oxygen, carbon dioxide, nutrients
Wetting of the anterior corneal surface
Maintenance of optical transparency
Optical correction of corneal surface irregularities
Disposal of foreign bodies
Defense against infection

Table **30**   Causes of tear deficiency
Dry environment: automobile, airplane, workplace
Hormone treatment (oral contraceptives, thyroxine, cortisone)
Pregnancy, nursing
Rheumatic diseases (Sjögren syndrome)
Aging, degeneration of the lacrimal glands
Chronic conjunctivitis
Thyroid and parathyroid disorders
Antibiotic treatment
Chronic infections, immune deficiency
Febrile illness
Diabetes mellitus, renal failure, adrenal dysfunction
Incomplete lid closure, malformed lids
Wearing contact lenses

Tear deficiency syndrome and its chief symptom, dry eye, have become increasingly common in recent years, particularly among contact lens wearers. The commonest cause of chronic conjunctivitis, it is a problem frequently encountered in the contact lens clinic. The causes of tear deficiency syndrome are listed in Table **30**; its increased frequency today is partly explained by greater levels of environmental pollution and stress, and by longer life expectancy.

Tear deficiency syndrome in a contact lens wearer should not be written off as a normal response to environmental pollution or as a psychosomatic manifestation requiring no treatment. Most patients experiencing discomfort with their contact lenses in fact have a demonstrable abnormality of tear function. Nor are the ill effects of tear deficiency syndrome limited to subjective discomfort: any quantitative or qualitative disturbance of the tear fluid can cause metabolic damage to the anterior segment. Absolute lack of tear fluid causes very severe trophic changes of the lids, conjunctiva, and cornea.

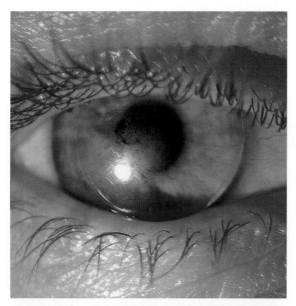

Fig. **426**   Dry eye in a wearer of hard contact lenses, dull lens surface, relative tear deficiency, qualitative deficit, wetting problem.

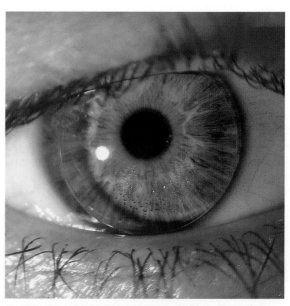

Fig. **427**   Dry eye in a wearer of hard contact lenses, air bubbles in the tear lens, quantitative tear deficit.

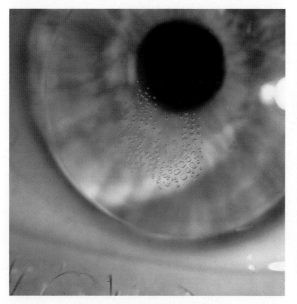

Fig. **428**   Dry eye in a wearer of hard contact lenses, air bubbles under the contact lens, quantitative tear deficit.

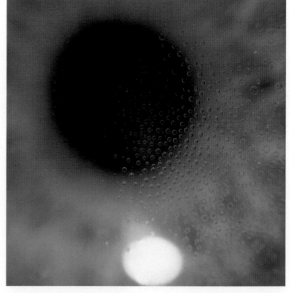

Fig. **429**   Dry eye in a wearer of hard contact lenses, bubbles in the tear lens from steep fitting, relative quantitative tear deficit.

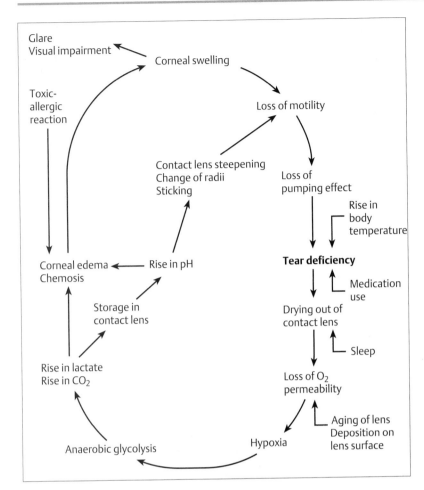

Illustration 10 Impairment of corneal metabolism by tear deficiency in the contact lens wearer. Tear deficiency leads to elevation of the temperature of the anterior corneal surface and thus to drying out of the contact lens, which thereby becomes less permeable to oxygen (lower Dk). The cornea is then forced to switch to anaerobic glycolysis, as a result of which lactate and pyruvate build up in the tear fluid. Corneal edema ensues, which further impairs lens motility, blocking exchange of the tear film and completing the vicious circle of corneal metabolic decompensation.

Tear deficiency in contact lens wearers promotes recurrent infection of the anterior ocular segment with impairment of vision, as well as drying out and sticking of the contact lenses and—mainly in soft hydrophilic lenses—a change in their refractive power. Protracted tear deficiency leads to a collapse of corneal metabolism by a vicious-circle mechanism, as illustrated in Illustration **10**. Thus, any clinically documented tear deficiency in a contact lens wearer requires prompt treatment, which should include the elimination of exogenous irritants, endogenous stimulation of lacrimation, reconstitution of a patent tear passageway if necessary, and/or substitution of tear fluid with a suitable artificial tear solution.

Clinical Course

The tear deficiency syndrome often develops gradually over several years and may be misdiagnosed at first, as its symptomatic presentation is more variable than that of many other ophthalmological conditions. At first, patients usually complain only of itching, burning, and the need to rub the eyes. The patient's report that the lids are stuck together in the morning and difficult to open is often the first indication of a disturbance of tear function. The foreign body sensation becomes progressively intense as contact lenses are worn, and visual problems develop, such as reduced contrast or increased glare. The patient must blink much more frequently. If tear deficiency syndrome in its early stages is not treated, or treated by the patient himself in unsupervised fashion with nonprescription eye drops, chronic conjunctivitis may ensue.

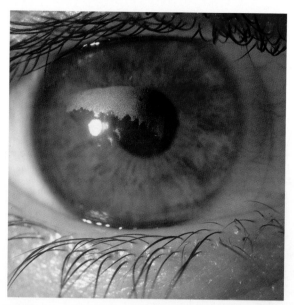

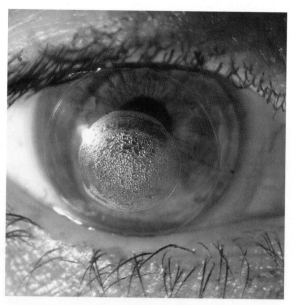

Fig. **430** Dry eye in a wearer of soft contact lenses, wetting problem, mucin deficiency, transient central clouding after each blink.

Fig. **431** Tear deficiency, piggyback system, deficit of aqueous phase, inadequate tear lens under a hard contact lens.

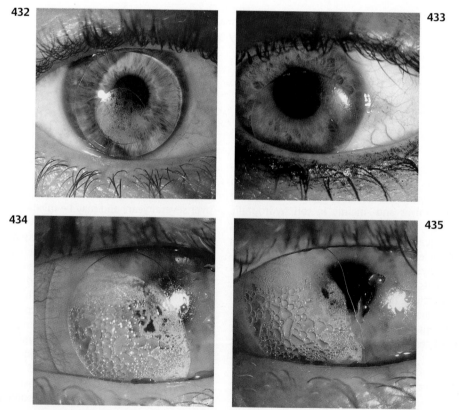

Fig. **432** Dry eye, hard contact lens, air bubble under the lens, deficit of aqueous phase.

Fig. **433** Dry eye, hard contact lens, hydrophobic lens surface, mucin deficiency.

Fig. **434** Tear deficiency, soft contact lens, drying evident after 8 hours of wear, bubbles under the lens.

Fig. **435** Tear deficiency, soft contact lens, bubbles under the lens after 8 hours of wear, surface wetting problem.

436

437

438

439

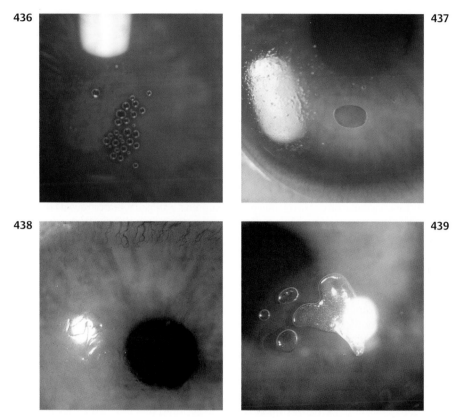

Fig. **436** Tear deficiency, soft contact lens, collection of bubbles under the lens, epithelial damage.

Fig. **437** Dried out soft lens, bubble under the lens, poor wetting of the lens surface.

Fig. **438** Tear deficiency. Dried out, deformed soft lens of high water content.

Fig. **439** Tear deficiency. Dried out, deformed soft lens of high water content, bubbles under the lens, epithelial lesion.

Whenever patients report discomfort while wearing contact lenses, and particularly when there is recurrent or chronic infection of the anterior ocular segment, the tear fluid should be both qualitatively and quantitatively assessed. The suspected diagnosis of tear deficiency syndrome can be confirmed by a simple test: test application of a drop of artificial tear solution in the lower cul-de-sac causes immediate resolution of the foreign body sensation and visual disturbance, which reappear after a variable interval (minutes to hours).

Dry eye can be worsened by air conditioning or by heating, particularly in an enclosed space such as an automobile. The eyes and contact lenses dry out rapidly in such situations. At first, visual acuity is little affected, but glare is increased. Dry eyes in the contact lens wearer are often accompanied by mild lid swelling and by bulbar conjunctival injection near the limbus at the 3-o'clock and 9-o'clock position, which may be grossly visible. The symptoms and signs of tear deficiency in the contact lens wearer are listed in Table **31**.

Hard contact lenses, if examined while still on the eye in tear deficiency syndrome, show a dull surface with dry areas, possibly with adherent remnants of pigment from eye make-up. Soft lenses have plaques and may be deformed; changes of the central corneal curvature are best detected with an ophthalmometer or keratometer. Visual acuity is decreased and is not improved by over-refraction, yet transiently normalizes upon instillation of artificial tears in the lower cul-de-sac.

Slit-lamp examination always reveals evidence of acute or chronic conjunctivitis, that is, diffuse, brick-red bulbar conjunctival hyperemia, possibly accompanied by bulbar conjunctival folds parallel to the lid margin.

The gross appearance of the cornea is normal, but fluorescein staining reveals sporadic, fine, stippled epithelial defects, which (like conjunctival hyperemia) are somewhat more pronounced along the horizontal than along the vertical axis.

In mild cases, fluorescein staining after lens removal shows no more than a barely detectable corneal edema. In more severe cases, cellular metaplasia and other defects are present and readily visible with rose bengal staining, and pachymetry reveals that the dried-out cornea is somewhat thinner than normal.

Decompensated tear deficiency syndrome in the contact lens wearer is characterized by multiple epithelial defects, stromal swelling, and endothelial changes, all of which indicate a collapse of corneal metabolism. There may be clinical progression to chronic conjunctivitis or tight lens syndrome (TLS).

In the most severe cases, tear deficiency may lead to keratitis; when tears are totally absent, as in lagophthalmic keratitis, corneal ulceration may occur, leading to permanent corneal damage and loss of visual function. Type B keratoconus also seems to have a causal relationship to tear deficiency, as a significant tear deficiency is always present in the early stage of the disease.

The symptoms of tear deficiency syndrome are more pronounced in contact lens wearers than in spectacle wearers, because the comfort of contact lens wear essentially depends on the presence of adequate tear fluid. A dry, dull lens surface, air bubbles between the lens and the cornea after long periods of wear, and immobility of the lens during blinking or saccadic movements are sure signs of tear deficiency or inadequate wetting. Fluctuating refractive power, or instability of the cylinder axis, in wearers of soft lenses also indicates that the lens is not fully moistened by the tear fluid.

Table **31** Symptoms of tear deficiency in contact lens wearers
Foreign body sensation
Eye-rubbing
Burning
Itching
Visual impairment
Glare
Reduced contrast
Haloes, veiled vision
Deformation of gel contact lenses

440

441

442

443

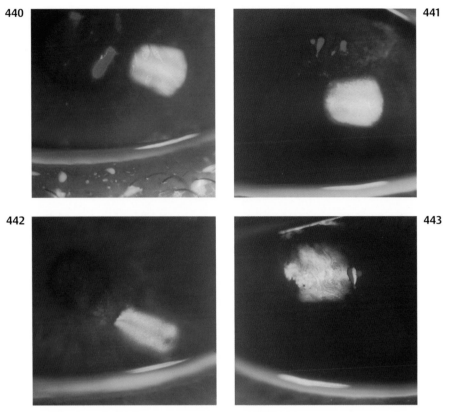

Fig. **440** Corneal erosion in a soft lens wearer with tear deficiency, diminished corneal reflex from drying.

Fig. **442** Corneal edema and epithelial damage due to tear deficiency, hard contact lens, deficit of aqueous phase.

Fig. **441** Corneal erosion, incipient bullous separation, tear-deficient soft lens wearer, diminished corneal reflex caused by drying of the corneal surface.

Fig. **443** Epithelial and stromal edema due to tear deficiency, hard contact lens, deficit of the wetting component of tears.

444

445

446

447

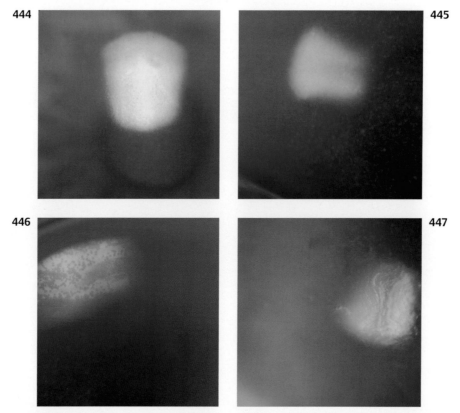

Fig. **444** Decreased slit-lamp reflex from the anterior surface of a soft contact lens, inadequate wetting of the lens material.

Fig. **446** Poor wetting, instability of the tear film on the anterior surface of a hard lens, mucin deficiency.

Fig. **445** Decreased slit lamp reflex from the anterior surface of a soft contact lens, staining shows stippling of the lens surface, lens desiccated.

Fig. **447** Poor wetting, instability of the tear film on the anterior surface of a soft lens.

448

449

450

451

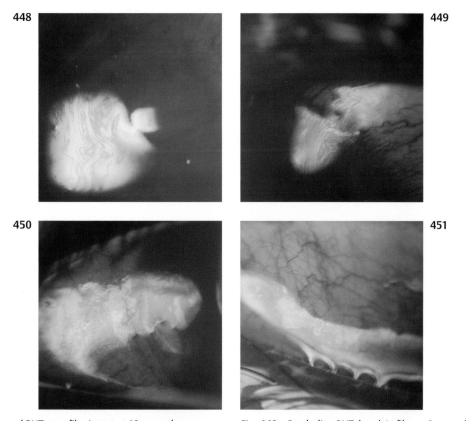

Fig. **448** Normal BUT: tear film intact at 10 seconds.

Fig. **449** Borderline BUT, break in film at 8 seconds.

Fig. **450** Pathological BUT, break in film at 5 seconds.

Fig. **451** Highly pathological BUT, break in film at 2 seconds.

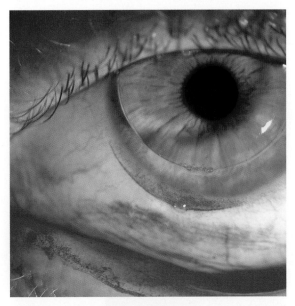

Fig. **452** Tear deficiency, hard contact lens, rose bengal staining, abrasion below the limbus caused by the lens because of tear deficiency.

453

454

455

456

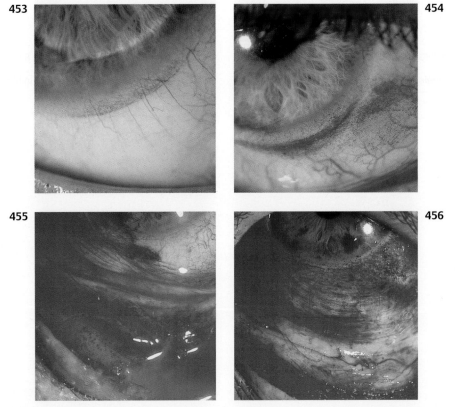

Fig. **453** Perilimbal traces of abrasion from wearing hard contact lenses, relative tear deficiency, staining with rose bengal.

Fig. **455** Hard lens wearer with severe tear deficiency, absolutely unable to wear contact lenses.

Fig. **454** Traces of abrasion from the overlying hard contact lens, tear deficiency, rose bengal staining.

Fig. **456** Severe tear deficiency syndrome, absolute contraindication for contact lenses.

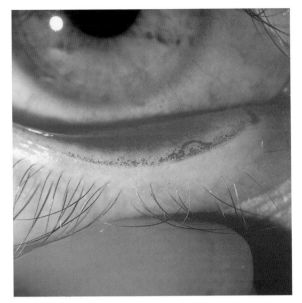 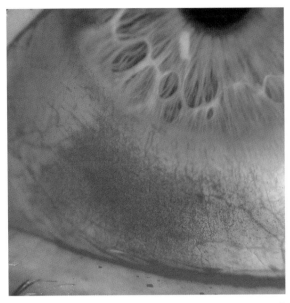

Fig. **457** Tear deficiency, rose bengal test after 8 hours of wearing a RGP lens.

Fig. **458** Tear dysfunction, soft contact lens wearer, traces of conjunctival abrasion, rose bengal staining.

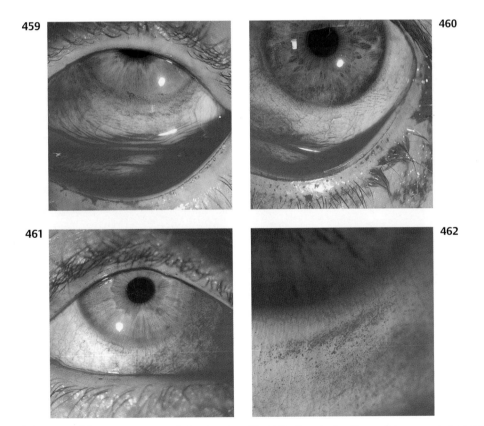

Fig. **459** Tear deficiency, soft lens wearer, traces of abrasion at the limbus, rose bengal staining.

Fig. **460** Tear dysfunction, soft lens wearer, traces of abrasion on the cornea and conjunctiva, rose bengal staining.

Fig. **461** Tear deficiency, soft lens wearer, traces of abrasion in the region covered by the lens haptic, rose bengal staining.

Fig. **462** Corneoscleral lens wearer with dry eye, conjunctival epithelial lesions with marked staining at the limbus, poor fitting, loss of lens.

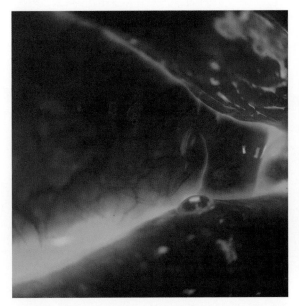

Fig. **463** Dry eye, aphakia, tear deficiency syndrome. Lens worn without difficulty after insertion of a flow-controller in the lower punctum.

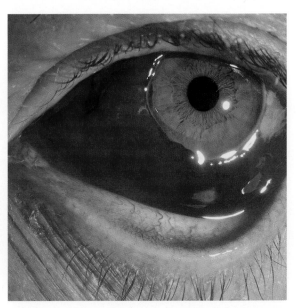

Fig. **464** Blunt trauma from a squash ball in a wearer of soft lenses.

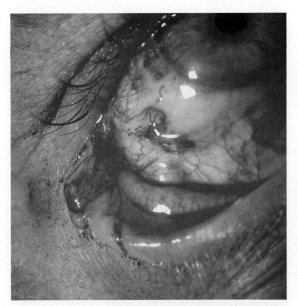

Fig. **465** Perforating wound from a screwdriver; RGP lens wearer.

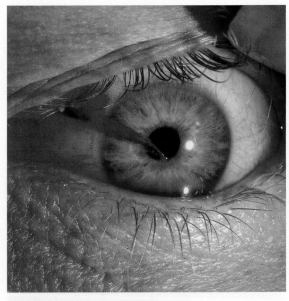

Fig. **466** Perforating wound from a glass shard; soft contact lens wearer.

Clinical Testing

The diagnosis of tear deficiency syndrome is established by quantitative and qualitative clinical testing of tear function. Testing is difficult in routine practice, however, because of the small volumes concerned, as compared to other bodily secretions: the average normal daily production of tear fluid is only about 1.0 ml. Thus, tear deficiency syndrome cannot always be reliably diagnosed in its early stage.

A single test does not suffice to establish the diagnosis of tear deficiency, as there may be an isolated disturbance of the volume of tear production or of wettability, and there are also combined disorders that cannot be reliably diagnosed with the Schirmer test or by measurement of the break-up time (BUT). Therefore, when there is clinical suspicion of tear deficiency syndrome, the use of multiple tests of the types described here is recommended. The more important tests are listed in Tables **32** and **33**.

Schirmer I and II Tests

The simplest way to estimate the amount of tear flow is by the Schirmer I test (without local anesthetic) and the Schirmer II test (with a local anesthetic such as proparacaine), which, however, like most other methods of direct measurement, provide only an inexact estimate of the total secreted volume. All direct methods elicit reflex tearing through contact with sensitive tissue, and may thus yield artificially high values; on the other hand, the relative hypesthesia induced by contact lens wearing sometimes diminishes reflex lacrimation, leading to artificially low values. Contact lenses must not be worn for at least 24 hours before the test. A normal finding in Schirmer I or Schirmer II is wetting of at least 10 mm of the test strip in 5 minutes.

Measurement of Break-up Time

The quality of the tear film is most easily assessed while the lens is on the eye by measurement of the lens tear-film BUT, which, unlike BUT measurement in the eye without a contact lens, is best performed without fluorescein. After spontaneous opening of the lids, the tear film on the anterior surface of the contact lens must remain intact for at least 10 seconds before breaking up. Values of 6–9 seconds are considered possibly abnormal; values less than 6 seconds are definitely abnormal and contraindicate the wearing of either hard or soft lenses for cosmetic reasons.

Meniscus Test

Measurement of the height of the tear meniscus at the center of the lower lid is performed with a reticle in one of the slit lamp eyepieces and, like BUT measurement, requires no contact with the anterior ocular segment. It is easily carried out during routine follow-up examination of the contact lens wearer. The result may, however, be difficult to interpret: values less than 0.2 mm are clearly abnormal, but higher values do not rule out tear deficiency syndrome, as dryness of the eye may be masked in the examining situation by reflex tearing.

Rose Bengal Test

Staining with a 2% solution of the vital dye rose bengal provides a much more accurate assessment of the state of the anterior ocular segment in dry eye syndrome. This test is primarily useful in advanced stages of the condition, as it stains necrotic epithelial cells; it is typically positive only when the Schirmer II test result is less than 3 mm and the BUT is less than 6 seconds. The contact lens must be removed before the dye is instilled in the inferior cul-de-sac, as it may otherwise be irreversibly stained. The dye is irritating, but the eye should not be pretreated with local anesthetic as this may produce false-positive results.

Lissamine Green Test

Like rose bengal, this dye stains necrotic epithelial cells, with the advantage that it does not sting.

Table **32** Recommended tests for the diagnosis of tear deficiencies
Schirmer I test
Schirmer II test (with local anesthetic)
BUT
Warm air provocation test
Fluorescein staining
Rose bengal staining
Meniscus test
Pachymetry
Thermometry

Table **33** Recommended blood tests in the diagnostic evaluation of tear deficiency
Iron
Sodium
Potassium
Calcium
Immunoglobulins
Rheumatoid factors
Blood glucose

Warm Air Provocation Test

This is a simple and easy provocative test for dry eye in the contact lens wearer. A stream of warm air from an electric hair drier is directed at the patient's open eyes from a distance of 1 m. Patients complaining of an uncomfortable foreign body sensation or dryness within 10 seconds usually suffer from a tear disorder.

Pachymetry

Pachymetry and (better still) micropachymetry are the most accurate diagnostic tests for tear deficiency syndrome in contact lens wearers and enable differentiation of its various stages and clinical types. The central corneal thickness (CCT) is normally $545 \pm 20\,\mu m$. Values less than 525 μm indicate thinning of the cornea through desiccation, tissue loss, or both; in such cases, the average CCT over the course of the day is below 500 μm. On the other hand, absolute or near-absolute lack of tears can cause marked corneal swelling, to a CCT well over 600 μm. When interpreting CCT values, however, one must remember that the corneal thickness is subject to the influence of various mechanical and metabolic factors when contact lenses are worn. It is therefore advisable to measure the CCT several times over the course of the day. Another, easier way to test for tear deficiency syndrome is to measure the CCT before and after instillation of a drop of artificial tear fluid in the conjunctival sac; if the CCT remains constant over the ensuing 20 minutes, then tear function is adequate.

Thermometry

Measuring the temperature of the anterior segment is a further aid to the diagnosis of tear deficiency syndrome. Infrared thermography of the cornea and conjunctiva provide the clearest documentation of temperature changes, but it requires specialized equipment that is not usually available in routine clinical practice. Instead, the temperature of the anterior segment can be measured with a hand-held thermistor placed on the fold of the closed upper lid. The normal temperature is 35–36°C; elevations are due to relative or absolute tear deficiency. This method can be used to assess the efficacy of treatment for dry eye with eye drops, gels, sprays, or ointments: the longer the decline in temperature persists after one of these products is applied, the more effective the treatment.

Note: The cause of dry eye should be determined before treatment is initiated; underlying disease processes, if found, should be treated first. Artificial tears should be used as little as possible, in order not to suppress lacrimation. Gels and ointments are contraindicated while contact lenses are worn.

Other Eye Diseases

The wearing of contact lenses is contraindicated when topical medications must be applied for a shorter or longer time for the treatment of any disease of the outer or inner portion of the eye, such as glaucoma or iritis. The wearing of contact lenses may also be problematic in the postoperative setting, for example after operations for strabismus or cataract, after surgical creation of a fistula for glaucoma, or after retinal reattachment. Postoperative scars, infections, and trauma may interfere with the wearing of contact lenses. The particular problems associated with lens fitting after surgical creation of a fistula for glaucoma are discussed in another chapter of this book (see p. 201).

The above conditions are not an absolute contraindication to the wearing of contact lenses for refractive or cosmetic indications, but they do lead to more frequent complications. If contact lenses are to be worn, frequent ophthalmologic follow-up is mandatory.

The above conditions are sometimes themselves treated with therapeutic contact lenses. In such cases, special ophthalmological and fitting techniques are required, for example the additional administration of various types of therapeutic eye drops.

8 Eye Injuries in Contact Lens Wearers

Types of Ocular Trauma

Trauma Involving Foreign Bodies

Perforated Globe

Ocular Contusion

Chemical Injury

Consequences for Contact Lens Wearers

Types of Ocular Trauma

Eye injuries account for some 2–3% of all injuries of the human body and are most often due to the direct or indirect effect of foreign bodies, liquids, or gases on the eye, usually as the result of an accident. Such injuries are about equally frequent in persons who wear contact lenses, spectacles, or neither.

Emergency visits to the general ophthalmologist or to the contactologist are usually due to foreign-body or chemical injuries. Relatively efficient protection against injuries of these types is afforded by spectacles, even better protection by goggles that are worn in the workplace where there would otherwise be a risk of eye injury. The contact lens wearer, however, cannot benefit from the protective function of spectacles, and all too often disregards medical advice to wear protective goggles in those situations where they are indicated.

> **Note:** Many contact lens wearers neglect to wear protective goggles in the mistaken idea that contact lenses themselves protect the eye. No chance should be missed to correct this error. Contact lenses do not protect the eye either against foreign bodies, or against very bright light (e.g., in welding).

Trauma Involving Foreign Bodies

Unlike spectacles or goggles, contact lenses do not protect the eyes against metallic shards expelled in projectile fashion from lathes, grinders, planing machines, or other types of apparatus. Slit-lamp examination reveals the shards embedded in the contact lens as well as in areas of the conjunctiva and cornea not covered by it.

Glowing hot shards from welding can become embedded in the matrix of the lens, leaving visible tracks; they can even pierce soft lenses. Metallic particles embedded in a hydrophilic contact lens may rust and render the lens unwearable.

Just as dangerous are wooden splinters ejected from grinders, lathes, circular saws, and milling machines. These organic splinters often serve as a vehicle for bacteria and fungi that can attack both the eye and the contact lens.

Explosives and firecrackers may cause irreversible eye injury, driving tiny bits of shrapnel into the lids, conjunctiva, cornea, and contact lens. Destruction of the lens surface is easily seen under the slit lamp or microscope. Lenses damaged in this way are unwearable, among other reasons because the foreign material embedded in them can chemically irritate the lids, conjunctiva, and cornea and cause further injury.

Perforated Globe

Open-globe injuries in contact lens wearers are often caused by fragments of a shattered windshield when the patient has been the unrestrained driver, or front-seat passenger, in an automobile accident. Such injuries can be very severe; on occasion, the contact lens must be surgically removed from the interior of the eye along with the glass shards. Goggles worn at the workplace do not afford 100% protection: We have seen a case in which a steel rod propelled from a machinist's lathe shattered his goggles, creating glass shards that destroyed his contact lens (worn because of aphakia) and simultaneously perforated the globe.

Ocular Contusion

Blunt trauma poses particular dangers for contact lens wearers. As an example, patients who wear spectacles can be injured by a flying tennis or squash ball only if its momentum is sufficient to shatter the spectacles and drive the shards into the eye. Contact lens wearers, however, lack the degree of protection that spectacles afford. If the flying object impacts against the contact lens or the globe, hemorrhage can result; in rare cases, the contact lens is shattered.

We have seen a case in which a flying champagne cork directly impacted against a rigid contact lens, not shattering it, but deforming it so that it had to be replaced. In fact, contact lenses must be replaced whenever they are damaged by contact with a foreign body, even if the damage is small and confined to the edge of the lens. Tiny edge defects can cause ring-shaped conjunctival hemorrhage or circular corneal erosions if the lens continues to be worn. Moreover, such lenses, if worn, can produce pseudoherpetic corneal epithelial defects that are very difficult to distinguish from dendritic keratitis. If this situation should arise, the correct diagnosis can be made by careful inspection of the posterior surface of the lens.

Chemical Injury

Symptoms: Exogenous toxic chemicals induce marked acute conjunctival injection and chemosis, as well as corneal swelling. Other symptoms are pain and lid spasms that become more severe when the contact lenses are removed.

Clinical findings: Chemical injuries produce the same symptoms and have the same sequelae in contact lens wearers as in persons who do not wear contact lenses.

Not only solid foreign bodies, but also liquids splashed into the eye can damage the eye and contact lens. Now and again, contact lens wearers, mistakenly thinking that they are wearing spectacles, spray an eyeglass-cleaning solution directly into a contact-lens-bearing eye. Hard lenses are rarely damaged in such incidents, but soft lenses may store the detergent chemicals in the cleaning solution and later re-release them into the eye, causing severe irritation. Thus, whenever eyeglass-cleaning solution is sprayed onto a contact lens, the lens should be discarded.

We have encountered another case in which inadvertent switching of cosmetics resulted in the application of fingernail polish containing silver particles to the eyelids. Some of the silver particles found their way onto the conjunctiva, cornea, and contact lens, destroying the lens.

Accidents with gaseous substances occur in the workplace and elsewhere. Many water-soluble gases can be taken up by contact lenses and then severely irritate the eye when they are re-released during contact lens wear; examples include tear gas, CS gas, and pepper spray. Firemen are often exposed to chemical fumes that can be taken up by soft lenses, causing discoloration and deformation of the lens and deposition on its surface. Contact lenses that have been involved in such incidents should be destroyed.

Peroxide injuries are, unfortunately, common in contact lens wearers. They are usually the result of inadvertent switching of solutions, so that the lens is stored in the neutralizing solution and then rinsed in hydrogen peroxide. A contributory cause of such accidents is inadequate instruction of the patient regarding the use of lens hygiene products and the dangers of misuse. This only underscores the need for thorough patient instruction.

Consequences for Contact Lens Wearers

Any cut, burn, or chemical injury to the eye of a contact lens wearer requires immediate ophthalmological examination and treatment. The contact lens should be removed at once and its inner and outer surfaces inspected under the microscope. The eye must be carefully examined to assess the nature and extent of injury. Fluorescein staining should be performed to detect any possible epithelial injury.

> **Note:** Contact lens wearers must be made aware that contact lenses have no protective function. Contact lenses can absorb dangerous fluids and gases of many different kinds and can be destroyed by a wide variety of mechanical or chemical influences. Whenever the eye is injured, the lens should be removed from the eye as soon as possible. The patient often has difficulty doing this himself because of the accompanying lid spasm. This alone would be sufficient reason for any contact lens wearer with an eye injury, or even the suspicion of one, to seek ophthalmological assistance immediately.

9 Frequency of Contact Lens Complications

Analysis of Contact Lens Complications

Analysis of Contact Lens Complications

Contact lens complications and their frequency of occurrence have been the subject of many published reports; the most important ones are listed in Table **34**. Estimates of frequency vary markedly across the international literature because of the lack of uniform standards of definition or assessment. Some authors report complication rates as high as 30%, depending on the variety of lens, lens care system, and mode of wear, while others report complication rates well under 1%. Any such figure should be viewed critically, as most reports fail to state either the composition of the patient population or the length of wearing time.

It is clear, however, that an accurate quantitative estimate of risk would be of great use to manufacturers, fitters, and, above all, patients. In our analysis, we divide contact lens complications into two groups, as shown in Tables **35** and **36**: those that occur in the first year of wear, and those that typically occur only after 10 or more years of wear. These two types of complication show very different statistical behavior.

Distinguishing in this way between initial and long-term contact lens complications provides useful information for the development of new lens materials and lens care products and the improvement of those already in use. Once contact lenses have been worn successfully for 1 year, the likelihood of a complication becomes much lower, as the patient's handling of the lenses improves with experience and allergic reactions have usually been eliminated by the end of the first year by a change of lens material or lens care products, if necessary. On the other hand, any intractable problems of handling or allergy that may arise usually result in a reversion to spectacles or other visual aids within the first year. Interestingly, patients who wear contact lenses for medical reasons and have no viable therapeutic alternative to them seem to tolerate their lenses much better than those who wear them for refractive correction, who can always fall back on spectacles if desired.

Many problems and complications of contact lens wear can be prevented by the identification of possible hindrances and risk factors before the lenses are fitted (see p. 160). All too frequently, contraindications to contact lens wear are overlooked or disregarded at the fitting stage, and later, when the patient has begun to wear the lenses. The resulting difficulties may later cause not only frustration for the fitter and the patient, but also severe, irreversible eye damage. Problems of this type are the most common cause of malpractice suits against contact lens fitters.

The potential risk factors that must be taken into account are numerous and by no means limited to ocular pathology; systemic problems such as an allergic predisposition, immune deficiency, or metabolic disease often complicate contact lens wear. Medication use, too, including the use of oral contraceptives, may complicate contact lens wear by an effect on the composition of the tear fluid. Low patient intelligence or generally negligent personal grooming are predictors of faulty lens handling and hygiene. Even the suspicion of poor patient compliance with the recommendations for proper lens care is a sufficient contraindication for contact lens fitting. Problems of this nature are, of course, not restricted to the wearing of contact lenses, but are found in all fields of medicine.

The most common causes of contact lens complications, and their frequencies, are listed in Table **37**. As can

Table **36**   Contact lens complications that generally arise only after years of wear
Corneal distortion syndrome
Endothelial changes
Stromal thinning
Neovascularization

Table **34**   The most common contact lens complications
Blepharospasm
Allergic blepharitis
Pseudoptosis
Giant papillary conjunctivitis (GPC)
Conjunctivitis simplex
Pseudoepiscleritis
Neovascularization
Toxic keratopathy
Corneal erosions, epithelial defects
Superficial keratitis
Overwear syndrome
Corneal deprivation syndrome (CDS)
Tight lens syndrome (TLS)
Corneal ulcer
Panophthalmitis

Table **35**   Contact lens complications in the first year of wear
Disinfectant allergy
Injury due to faulty insertion and removal
Injury due to faulty lens handling
Infections of the lids, conjunctiva, and cornea
Toxic keratopathy
Injury due to material defects and manufacturing errors

be seen from the table, approximately three-quarters of all complications are due to poor patient compliance. This underscores the fitter's vital responsibility to provide the patient with clear, thorough, and, when necessary, repeated instruction and counseling on proper lens care. Proper patient education cannot be assured if contact lenses are acquired by mail order or over the Internet.

Table **37** Causes and frequency of contact lens complications

Faulty handling	22%
Faulty cleaning	20%
Faulty disinfection	18%
Wearing time exceeded	15%
Secondary ocular disease	11%
Primary ocular disease	6%
Fitting errors	4%
Material errors	3%
Manufacturing errors	1%

10 Treatment of Contact Lens Complications

General Aspects

General Treatment Procedures

Special Treatment Procedures

Lid Diseases

Conjunctival Diseases

Scleral Diseases

Corneal Diseases

Intraocular Findings

Glaucoma

Dry Eye, Tear- Deficiency Syndrome

Accidents, Mechanical Trauma, Chemical Trauma

General Aspects

Contact lens complications can only be treated after their cause has been determined by a thorough ophthalmological examination. The type of treatment that could be provided is a function of the etiology, symptoms, physical findings, and severity of the problem. Some of the more common complications and medications often used to treat them are listed in Table **38**.

Table **38** Useful ophthalmic preparations in the treatment of contact lens complications

Blepharospasm	oxybuprocaine*
Blepharitis	gentamicin sulfacetamide/prednisolone fluocortolone
Pseudoptosis	zinc sulfate cromolyn sodium
Giant papillary conjunctivitis	Iodoxamide cromolyn sodium
Chemosis	dexamethasone
Conjunctivitis simplex	naphazoline phenylephrine
Pseudoscleritis	Iodoxamide
Vascularization	nandrolone diclofenac
Toxic keratopathy	cromolyn sodium nandrolone
Corneal erosion	erythromycin vitamin A/B_{12} calcium pantothenate
Superficial keratitis	ofloxacin gentamicin
Overwear syndrome	dexpanthenol calcium pantothenate
Corneal deprivation syndrome	vitamins
Tight lens syndrome	polyvinyl alcohol saline
Corneal ulceration	ofloxacin gentamicin pimaricin fusidic acid
Tear deficiency syndrome	artificial tear solutions

* For emergency treatment only

General Treatment Procedures

The first and most important step in the treatment of all contact lens complications is discontinuation of the contact lens. Whenever a complication is encountered or even suspected, the lens should be removed from the eye immediately and not reinserted until the cause of the problem has been determined and the eye has completely healed.

Removing the lens from the eye may be difficult in some emergency situations. The use of a local anesthetic may facilitate removal of the lens but may render the lens unwearable from that moment onward; moreover, all local anesthetics are relatively toxic to the eye and therefore unsuitable for use except in the short term. It is sometimes possible to remove a lens after application of only one or two drops of artificial tear or buffer solution, which causes the lens to float off the ocular surface so that it can be readily removed. This is the recommended method for removing stuck lenses in cases of tight lens syndrome (TLS) or overwear syndrome. Likewise, prior instillation of a few drops of a wetting solution is helpful when a lens must be removed from an anxious patient or a child.

Once a contact lens has been removed from the eye, its surface should be cultured, and it should be examined in the laboratory for defects and deposits. The lens should be meticulously cleaned and disinfected before it is returned to the patient, or else the original disease process—such as conjunctivitis or keratitis—may be reactivated. Unfortunately, patients often disregard medical advice and reinsert their lenses too soon after an injury or bout of infection, after inadequate disinfection, or when the lenses have been found to be defective. Any of these errors can reactivate the problem that necessitated removal of the lenses in the first place.

Once the lens has been removed, the second therapeutic step is the treatment of the problem in the eye, in accordance with standard ophthalmological practice. In the selection of medications, preservative-free eye drops and ointments are generally to be preferred, as wearers of contact lenses are at risk for a wide variety of complications related to the long-term effect of complex chemical compounds. These complications are due to interactions between the organic polymer structure of the lens material and the toxic or allergenic substances found in cleaning and disinfectant solutions, which have a chronic deleterious effect on the anterior ocular segment. Predictably, problems caused by any specific type of lens care product usually respond poorly to treatment with preparations containing the same type of preservative.

The length of time the patient must wait before reinserting the lens after the lesion has healed depends on the specific type of complication and its consequences for the eye. In general, after an ocular infection or traumatic lesion has healed, the contact lens should not be reinserted for at least 21 days. Severe complications, such as a corneal ulcer, require longer lens-free intervals, while, for a minor condition such as conjunctivitis, a few days will suffice.

> **Note:** The initial treatment of any contact lens complication is removal of the lens from the eye. Contact lens complications should never be treated with medications while the lens is still on the eye, except with artificial tears, if necessary. The lens can be removed from the eye with the aid of a normal saline solution if necessary, or with a local anesthetic if this does not work.

Special Treatment Procedures

Lid Diseases

Blepharospasm

Blepharospasm improves once its cause is diagnosed and eliminated. If it is due to mechanical irritation, it can be treated changing the contact lenses or the fitting concept, or by the regular use of artificial tears. The increased flow of tears associated with blepharospasm can be normalized more quickly, if necessary, with mildly astringent, soothing eye drops.

If blepharospasm impedes removal of a contact lens in an emergency situation, a local anesthetic can be given to eliminate it. A soft contact lens must be discarded after local anesthetic is used, because it can take up the anesthetic and re-release it to the eye, creating the risk of toxic keratopathy.

Ptosis

Ptosis is treated by elimination of its cause. If it is due to foreign-body irritation from the contact lens, it usually resolves without further treatment within a few days or, at most, weeks of the discontinuation of the lens, and requires no further treatment. If it is due to irritation of the tarsal conjunctiva, it can be eliminated by the instillation of mildly astringent eye drops.

Levator dysfunction is irreversible in rare cases after decade-long wearing of contact lenses. If the ptosis is cosmetically unacceptable or impairs vision, surgery can be performed to widen the palpebral fissure.

Lid Edema

Lid edema, too, is treated by elimination of its cause. The treatment of choice is calcium, given by the oral or (in extreme, acute cases) parenteral route, or sometimes cortisone in severe cases. Medical consultation should be obtained when lid edema does not seem to be related to the wearing of contact lenses, in which case a systemic illness may be responsible.

Squamous Blepharitis

Redness, swelling, and scaling of the lid margins imply intolerance to the contact lens material, lens care products, or other agents used in the eye. The possible causative substances include not only the cleaning and disinfecting solutions but also the wetting solutions that are often recommended to improve wearing comfort. Even eye ointments and drops that are used to treat contact lens complications can evoke an allergic response at the lid margin. The response usually takes the form of a classic squamous blepharitis. In many cases, squamous blepharitis that was present to some degree before the contact lenses were fitted is exacerbated by an allergic response to the contact lens or lens care solutions. The offending factor can sometimes be identified with a skin-prick test, but may be hard to eliminate, because such factors are both numerous and ubiquitous in the environment.

Before lid margin inflammation or ocular allergy is treated, the cause of the allergic diathesis should be identified, in consultation with a dermatologist if necessary, and the patient should refrain from wearing lenses until all symptoms and abnormal findings in the eye have resolved. Only then should the patient try to wear contact lenses again. A new lens material or new lens care system can be tried, possibly a peroxide-based system, as peroxide is not in itself allergenic.

Infectious and allergic lid problems should be treated with anti-inflammatory, antibiotic, and corticosteroid eye drops that are instilled three to four times daily, or, even better, an ointment applied to the affected areas two to three times daily. Multivalent mixed preparations are recommended. Salicylate eye baths improve comfort.

Lid Trauma

Traumatic lid injuries generally heal within a few days if the patient stops wearing contact lenses and applies re-epithelializing eye drops or ointment three to four times a day. Small cuts usually heal without treatment. Surgical intervention is needed to preserve lid function only for the rare larger or heavily bleeding wounds. In such cases, the preservation of an intact lid margin is very important, for otherwise the wearing of contact lenses may be problematic in future.

Antibiotic eye drops or ointment are used three to four times daily only for deeper injuries or where there is a risk of bacterial infection. Daily or twice-daily eye baths with a 1% salicylate solution improve comfort.

Conjunctival Diseases

Giant Papillary Conjunctivitis

The treatment of giant papillary conjunctivitis (GPC) is often unsatisfactory. Papillary hypertrophy regresses slowly and is sometimes present weeks after the patient has stopped wearing lenses. Cortisone is of no benefit. Most eye drops contain preservatives and only worsen the condition by denaturing the proteins normally found in the tear fluid, leading to further irritation.

The only treatment that has proved useful to date is with 2–3% cromolyn sodium or lodoxamide eye drops, instilled two to five times a day, just as in vernal conjunctivitis (a disorder of related etiology). At least 3 weeks and sometimes as long as 3 months of treatment will be required, and contact lenses should not be worn during this time. If the contact lenses are medically indicated and cannot be discontinued (e.g., in keratoconus), then the first daily dose of the preparation should be given early in the morning, at least 15 or 20 minutes before the lenses are inserted. One or two further doses should be given at midday, during a short lens-free interval, and the last dose in the evening, after the lens is removed. These measures prevent interaction of the medication with the lens material.

Patients who wear contact lenses while being treated for GPC should always remove and clean their lenses after 4–6 hours of wear and wait 20–30 minutes before reinserting them. This should prevent the lenses from becoming spoiled. If GPC should flare up again when the lenses are reinserted, the lens material should be changed immediately to avoid a full-blown recurrence. Furthermore, once GPC has resolved, the lens care system should be changed. In light of the complex etiology of GPC, a preservative-free system is generally preferred.

Conjunctival Chemosis

Acute chemosis must be treated immediately, whatever its cause. The conjunctiva should be rinsed immediately with corticosteroid eye drops, which the patient should then continue to instill every 1–2 hours during waking hours. The chemosis then usually resolves within 1 day. Only rarely is a Passow operation under local anesthesia necessary to restore lid function when chemosis interferes with lid closure.

It is important to be sure that the cortisone drops do not contain the same preservative agent that precipitated the problem. The use of unit-dose, preservative-free eye drops or ointment is recommended.

Conjunctival Hemorrhage

Mechanically induced conjunctival hemorrhage is characterized by a focal, circumscribed injury of the superficial conjunctival vessels and generally requires no treatment other than discontinuation of the contact lens until the lesion is healed. The same is true of small hemorrhagic conjunctival erosions caused by faulty lens insertion or removal or by the wearing of defective lenses. Eye drops should not be used; instead, healing and re-epithelializing ointments can be applied 3–4 times daily.

Extensive conjunctival hemorrhages in contact lens wearers are treated just as in other patients. Re-epithelializing and soothing ointments or gels are sufficient treatment for all but the largest hemorrhages. In rare cases of persistent bleeding, treatment by laser, cautery, or suture under local anesthesia may be required.

Heparin-containing ointments promote the resorption of conjunctival hemorrhages. If hemorrhage has occurred in the setting of therapeutic anticoagulation, it may be advisable to interrupt this treatment for a few days after consultation with the internist.

Conjunctival Trauma

Conjunctival trauma in contact lens wearers is generally treated just as in other patients. Contact lens wear is temporarily discontinued, antibiotic ointment or eye drops are applied, and the lesions usually regress within a few days. The course of healing should be documented with frequent follow-up examinations because there may be coexistent contact-lens-induced microlesions of the corneal epithelium, which, if bacterial conjunctivitis should develop, can rapidly turn into a focus of superficial keratitis or a corneal ulcer.

The threat of corneal infection is even greater when resistant organisms are present. Thus, whenever infection occurs after injury of the anterior ocular segment, cultures of the eye, lens, and lens case must be performed, and the sensitivity spectrum of the pathogenic organisms determined.

Nonspecific Conjunctival Hyperemia

Conjunctival irritation of mechanical or metabolic origin is adequately treated by temporarily discontinuing the contact lens and instilling mildly astringent eye drops. Nonprescription vasoconstrictive agents, so-called "eye whiteners," should not be used, as they will mask the disease process and make it impossible to document improvement. Patients who disregard medical advice and use such preparations usually continue wearing their contact lenses as well.

Bacterial Conjunctivitis

Bacterial conjunctivitis in a contact lens wearer requires topical antibiotic treatment, as the pathogenic bacteria may otherwise spread and attack the chronically microtraumatized cornea, causing a corneal infiltrate or ulcer.

Because antibiotic resistance develops rapidly, and because treatment usually needs to be initiated before the culture results are available, we recommend treating conjunctivitis and keratitis in contact lens wearers with broad-spectrum antibiotic or gyrase-inhibitor eye drops or ointment. These should be applied every 2–3 hours, depending on severity.

Viral Conjunctivitis

The treatment of viral conjunctivitis in a contact lens wearer is usually directed against its cause. Mild cases are adequately treated with astringent eye drops, or, alternatively, with virustatic or virucidal agents. Bacterial superinfection, if present, necessitates combining these agents with an antibiotic.

Cortisone is useful in the treatment of severe cases of epidemic keratoconjunctivitis, but it should be used sparingly and only after exclusion of corneal herpes or other corneal lesions.

Fungal Conjunctivitis

Fungal conjunctivitis is difficult to treat, because few ophthalmic fungistatic or fungicidal preparations are available. These must be used three to four times daily for at least 3 weeks. The patient's immune status should be studied, as this type of infection generally arises in the setting of systemic illness or immune compromise.

Scleral Diseases

Scleral lesions in the contact lens wearer are treated in the same way as conjunctival lesions, according to their etiology. Soothing and anti-inflammatory ointments or eye drops may be used.

Corneal Diseases

Corneal Edema

Corneal edema in a contact lens wearer is treated by removing its cause, that is, the contact lens. Once lens wearing is discontinued, edema usually resolves within a few days. If it persists, it can be treated for a few days more with mildly astringent eye drops. Short-term use of nandrolone-containing, hyperosmolar, or buffered eye drops given locally two to three times a day speeds the healing process by restoring the osmotic stability of the cornea.

Corneal Erosion

Corneal epithelial defects are highly prone to recurrence and sometimes create a therapeutic problem because, once healed, they can reappear shortly after the patient resumes wearing contact lenses. The lenses should therefore not be reinserted until it is certain that the corneal epithelium has become firmly reanchored to the underlying tissue. This normally takes at least 3 weeks but may take much longer in contact lens wearers because of the chronic foreign-body irritation caused by the lens. If corneal erosion recurs, a therapeutic, gel "bandage" contact lens may be indicated.

Specific treatment for corneal erosion, beyond the temporary interdiction of contact lenses, is generally not required. The epithelial lesions usually disappear overnight after the lens is removed; it is only rarely necessary to treat for a few days with mildly astringent eye drops or ointment. When contact lens wearing is resumed, the lens material and lens care system should be of a new type.

Pseudoherpetic corneal erosions in contact lens wearers are best treated with re-epithelializing eye drops or ointment. Antibiotic ointment should be given locally in addition in case of bacterial superinfection.

A fresh corneal epithelial erosion can be treated with preparations that promote healing, such as dexpanthenol, or with antibiotics three to four times daily. Once the epithelium is fully healed, the instillation of nandrolone eye drops two to three times daily for 2–3 weeks will prevent recurrence.

Bullous Keratopathy

Bullous keratopathy is difficult to treat and frequently recurs. It seems reasonable to use astringent eye drops (in combination with a hyperosmolar preparation, if the stroma is involved). Therapeutic soft lenses can be useful as long as the lesion was not itself the result of a toxic reaction to a soft lens of the same type. If bullous keratopathy is caused purely by mechanical disruption of the epithelium in an otherwise healthy contact lens wearer, it will generally heal within 3–4 weeks after discontinuation of the contact lens and provision of re-epithelializing eye drops.

Tight Lens Syndrome

The initial step of treatment in tight lens syndrome is the removal of the adherent lens, with the aid of artificial tears or buffer solution if necessary to prevent corneal epithelial injury. If used, these eye drops should be instilled repeatedly at 5-minute intervals (just as in chemical burn injuries), until the lens no longer sticks to the cornea and moves with each blink. Antibiotic eye drops or ointment must be given locally for a few days thereafter, as this will help prevent corneal ulceration, a frequent complication of TLS.

Toxic Keratopathy

All forms of toxic keratopathy, and especially the very severe variety seen in mixed solution syndrome, mandate the immediate discontinuation of contact lenses, which should not be reinserted for several weeks or months.

There is no specific treatment for this condition. Cortisone is of no use in massive toxic reactions, and the preservatives found in most eye drop preparations tend to worsen the problem. Symptomatic relief can be gained by the use of astringent eye drops, such as a preservative-free 2% silver protein acetyl tannate solution applied three to four times daily; alternatives are corneal anabolic eye drops and cromolyn eye drops. In case of superinfection, preservative-free antibiotic preparations should be used.

Corneal Deprivation Syndrome

The discontinuation of contact lenses results in the regression of all contact-lens-induced metabolic disturbances, in particular those that result from an impaired delivery of vitamins and other essential substances to the cornea by way of the tear fluid. Corneal deprivation syndrome (CDS) results either from the depriving effect of lens materials of various types or from the increased metabolic demand of the cornea in contact lens wearers, or both; it usually resolves with no treatment besides removal of the lens. Complete healing usually requires discontinuation of the lens for 1–2 weeks, in severe cases as long as 3 weeks.

Corticosteroids and antibiotics do not accelerate healing, nor is the local application of nandrolone of any value. Hypertonic salt and glucose solutions are also of no use. Only the application of 1–2 drops of multivitamin and multi-amino-acid solution appears to help.

Post-heat Syndrome

The first step of treatment for post-heat syndrome is the immediate removal of the lenses, which generally requires instillation of a local anesthetic to counteract the associated blepharospasm. As in all chemical burns of the eye, buffering eye drops or ointment should be given repeatedly for the next 24–48 hours, and, if there is a tissue defect, antibiotics should be given as well. The contact lenses are no longer wearable and must be discarded. Allergy to the lens material should be ruled out before insertion of a new lens of the same type.

Keratitis, Corneal Infiltrates, Corneal Ulcers

The treatment of choice for bacterial keratitis or corneal ulceration in a contact lens wearer is the same as that used for bacterial conjunctivitis in persons who do not wear contact lenses: local application of high-dose antibiotic eye drops or ointment, with the selection of agent based on the pathogenic species and its spectrum of antibiotic sensitivity.

When treatment must be initiated before the culture results are available, as is usually the case, broad-spectrum antibiotic coverage is recommended with an agent such as gentamicin or a gyrase inhibitor. In the initial phase of treatment, antibiotic ointment should be applied every 1–2 hours (or eye drops every hour). The treatment must be continued for a minimum of 9 days; stopping earlier may lead to the breeding of resistant organisms, which then produce recurrent infection.

Acanthamoeba corneal ulceration in contact lens wearers is rare and difficult to treat. Current recommendations are for the local application of propamidine in combination with neomycin or polymyxin B; in severe cases, ketoconazole is given orally in addition. As in all deep infections of the cornea, mydriatics such as homatropine or scopolamine should be given concomitantly (after glaucoma has been excluded).

Corneal Vascularization

Corneal neovascularization as a complication of contact lens wear always regresses within a few months after the patient stops wearing contact lenses, leaving behind collapsed "ghost vessels," which require no treatment.

Contact-lens-induced corneal neovascularization is said to regress more rapidly if nandrolone-containing or astringent eyedrops are applied two or three times daily for a maximum of 6 weeks. On the other hand, the treatment of neovascularization into a transplanted cornea requires the local or even systemic administration of cortisone or immunosuppressive agents.

Should the patient wish to wear lenses in spite of corneal neovascularization, the fitting concept must be reviewed in the light of the factors that provoked the problem, and the lens must be changed to one made of material with a higher oxygen permeability (Dk) or a different chemical composition. If a toxic response to a lens care product is implicated in the causation of the problem, a new lens care product should be chosen that does not contain the offending substance.

Corneal Scars

Corneal scars may be treated conservatively in the same manner as corneal clouding of other causes, that is, with nonsteroidal anti-inflammatory agents or nandrolone, given in eye drop form three to four times daily for up to 4 weeks. Conservative management is often unsuccessful, however, and corneal scars that impair vision generally require surgery.

Corneal Deformation

There is no specific treatment for the restoration of a corneal contour that has been deformed by a contact lens; fortunately, the cornea usually returns to its original shape after the contact lens is discontinued. It has been claimed that the application of nandrolone eye drops two to three times daily can accelerate healing. In 80–90% of cases, the cornea returns to its original shape within 3 weeks; refraction for spectacles should be performed no earlier than this.

Folds in Descemet's Membrane, Endothelial Changes

Cortisone drops or local anabolic drops are useful in the treatment of folds in Descemet's membrane. Other endothelial changes do not regress, even after long periods of not wearing contact lenses. There is as yet no effective treatment that can stabilize the number of damaged endothelial cells or change their shape and size back to normal.

Intraocular Findings

Intraocular infection as a direct or indirect complication of contact lenses is treated with oral or parenteral antibiotics, with or without cortisone. It should be borne in mind that some types of antibiotics fail to enter the vitreous body or reach a therapeutically adequate intraocular concentration when they are given systemically. In addition to antibiotics, therapeutic mydriasis is a further important component of treatment.

Other types of intraocular process are nearly always unrelated to the wearing of contact lenses and require appropriate ophthalmologic evaluation and treatment. Depending on the form of treatment, it may be necessary for the patient to stop wearing lenses for a time.

Glaucoma

Glaucoma in contact lens wearers is treated in the same way as in other patients, and with the same objectives: Stabilization of the intraocular pressure and preservation of the visual field.

The dosage of antiglaucoma medication must be adjusted in contact lens wearers to account for alterations in pharmacodynamics caused by wearing contact lenses. A hard contact lens, for example, considerably prolongs the washout phase of medications delivered in eye drops, so that the quantity or concentration of the applied agent can be reduced by up to 50%.

A soft contact lens similarly prolongs washout and also has a storage effect, in that the hydrophilic lens material acts as a depot for all water-soluble substances. Thus, the concentration of eye drops used to treat glaucoma can be reduced to as little as 25% of the original concentration. No fixed rule can be given for the required adjustment in dose, as it depends on multiple factors, including the water content and mass of the lens and the specific agent used. In general, ionic lens materials take up the agent more readily than anionic materials and deliver it back to the tear fluid more slowly. In any contact-lens wearer, the proper dosage of antiglaucoma medication can only be determined by meticulous individual titration to the response of the intraocular pressure.

In patients with glaucoma who have undergone surgery to create a filtration bleb, the wearing of contact lenses poses the risk of acute injury to the bleb. While contact lenses are not considered to be absolutely contraindicated in this situation, the risks and benefits should be carefully weighed in each case.

Dry Eye, Tear Deficiency Syndrome

Tear deficiency in a contact lens wearer, if untreated, leads to a disturbance of the metabolism of the anterior ocular segment, with resulting complications. Thus, a dry eye in a contact lens wearer should be treated without delay. The results of treatment are often unsatisfactory: although there is a wide variety of artificial tear solutions available on the market, there is as yet no specific medication which, when given for a limited time, will permanently heal the dry eye of the contact lens wearer.

The form of treatment to be used in each patient depends on the particular cause of tear deficiency in that patient, and on the manifestations of tear deficiency syndrome that are found on ocular examination. Before initiating local treatment, the ophthalmologist should assess which endogenous and exogenous factors are responsible for tear deficiency in the individual patient. In unclear cases, medical consultation with an appropriate laboratory work-up is advisable.

An inadequate flow of tears to the eye must be diagnostically distinguished from a wetting disorder, as both types of disorder affect lens wearing comfort in a similar way. It should also be noted that the preservatives found in artificial tear solutions may be incompatible with the contact lens material.

The choice of wetting agent or artificial tear solution requires just as much care as, for example, that of an ophthalmic antibiotic or antiglaucoma agent. The danger of mixed solution syndrome must be borne in mind and averted, as toxic keratopathy may result if the artificial tear solution chosen is incompatible with the patient's lens care system. Preservative-free solutions are thus to be preferred, though even these should be used sparingly, as improper or excessive use of artificial tears has been shown to cause a significant reduction of the flow of the patient's own tear fluid.

For local therapy with eye drops there are certain basic guidelines: Salt deficiency is treated with hypertonic solutions, mucin deficiency with mucomimetic solutions. Eyes that are dry in the morning are treated with hyposmolar solutions to wash away the mucus that has accumulated overnight during sleep.

The osmolarity of the artificial tear solution should be chosen according to the central corneal thickness (CCT)—hypotonic solution for decreased CCT, hypertonic solution for increased CCT. In view of the problems caused by preservatives in artificial tear solutions, as mentioned above, long-term treatment is best provided with preservative-free solutions, for example, in unit-dose form.

The decision whether to treat dry eye with eye drops, a gel, or an ointment mainly depends on the frequency with which drops will have to be instilled, and on the lens-wearing regimen. A gel or ointment is preferable at times when the patient is not wearing contact lenses, e.g., during sleep, so that drops will not have to be instilled too frequently, although the patient may be bothered by the temporary impairment of vision that these preparations cause. Only eye drops can be used while the patient is wearing contact lenses.

Non-water-soluble medications delivered directly into the cul-de-sac are contraindicated while the patient is wearing contact lenses, as such substances can adhere to and damage the lenses. They can be used to restore the tear film only after the contact lenses have been removed, typically at night.

The proper dosage of medications for dry eye must be determined individually for each patient. Adequate relief for the entire day is often obtained from the instillation of a single drop of artificial tear solution in the morning upon awakening or from the use of a wetting solution during lens insertion. The optimal dosing schedule can only be determined by observing how long the patient is asymptomatic after the instillation of a single drop. The most common error in the treatment of dry eye in contact lens wearers is overdosing. If eyedrops are instilled too frequently, they interfere with the natural regulatory circuit of reflex-driven tear secretion and reduce the patient's own tear production, thereby worsening the condition they were supposed to treat.

Thus, the treatment for dry eye cannot be considered a routine matter. The eye drops that are chosen for the initial treatment must not be continually re-prescribed without follow-up; rather, the anterior ocular segment must be regularly re-examined to document the effect of treatment. In other words, the treatment of dry eye in a contact lens wearer requires just as much care as, for example, the treatment of glaucoma.

A new form of treatment for dry eye is the application of so-called dry-eye ointment once or twice daily to the lower lid, rather than in the conjunctival sac. The ease of use of this method is its main advantage, particularly for elderly patients. Recent research further suggests that dry eye in contact lens wearers can be efficiently treated with tear-stimulating substances delivered in liposomes in the form of a spray. A single application of spray results in pachymetric stabilization of the cornea and normalization of the elevated temperature of the anterior surface of the eye for up to 2 hours. This form of treatment commends itself for use in the workplace, as a single application of spray onto the closed eyelids can relieve symptoms for several hours.

If treatment with topical agents is unsuccessful, or if eye drops must be applied so frequently that the patient has trouble complying, then invasive treatment may be indicated as the next step, but only if the contact lenses must be worn for medical reasons, or if the use of other forms of visual aid is, for some reason, not possible. Partial occlusion of the lower punctum lacrimale with a silicone-tube flow controller and total blockage of tear outflow with a punctum plug are useful temporary treatments for tear deficiency syndrome that have largely replaced surgical procedures such as the irreversible closure of the lower punctum by cauterization.

Accidents, Mechanical Trauma, Chemical Trauma

Eye injuries in contact lens wearers should be treated according to the usual ophthalmological principles, with the addition that antibiotics should always be given, as the wearing of contact lenses confers a higher risk of post-traumatic infection.

After a chemical exposure, the contact lens must be safely removed before the eye is rinsed and treated with buffer solution in the usual fashion. Likewise, whenever ocular trauma is to be treated surgically, the ophthalmologist must first be sure to remove the contact lens, or any contact lens fragments, from the operative field.

In peroxide exposures, the lens must be removed from the eye at once, which may be difficult because of the painful blepharospasm. Copious rinsing with sterile isotonic saline (or, if this is unobtainable, with tap water) helps to dilute the offending chemical and wash it out of the eye. In the ideal situation, a neutralizing solution for peroxide is ready at hand; rinsing with it is the easiest and safest way to neutralize the offending chemical. Afterward, ointment is used to promote re-epithelialization. Larger epithelial defects require additional antibiotic coverage.

Note: Contact-lens-related complications (like any other ophthalmologic disorder) should be treated with one, or at most two, medications wherever possible, as the shot-gun approach can easily lead to mixed solution syndrome. Preparations that contain preservatives should be avoided for the same reason.

References

Alimgil ML, Erda N, Erda S, Aydinli J. Endothelial pathology in contact lens wearers. Contactologia. 1990;12E: 127–129.

Alimgil ML, Erda N, Gönenc D. Treatment of corneal disorders with bandage lenses. Contactologia. 1990;12E: 168–170.

Allansmith MR. The eye and immunology. St Louis:Mosby;1982.

Arrifin A. The cornea in diabetes. Contact Lens J.1992;20–14.

Asbell PA. Contact lens fitting after radial keratotomy and corneal transplant surgery. Contactologia. 1995;17E: 81–84.

Bale F, Rouland JF. Optical correction of post-traumatic juvenile aphakia. Contactologia. 1990;12E: 155–157.

Becker KW, Höh H. Histological changes in the porcine corneal following Nd: YAG laser keratotomy. Contactologia. 1990;12E: 13–21.

Behrens-Baumann W. Contact lenses and keratomycosis: a survey. Contactologia. 1993;15E: 41–43.

Beirnaert V, Haenens JD, Dhooge M, Brondel G, Passel van G. Photokeratometry—a review. Contactologia. 1991;13E: 81–89.

Bennet ES, Henry VA. Clinical Manual of contact lenses. Philidelphia:Lippincott;1994.

Bergmanson JP, Chu LW. Corneal response to rigid contact lens wear. Brit. J. Ophthalm.1982;66: 667–675.

Bialasiewicz A, Janssen K. Inflammatory disorders of the outer eye and anterior segment. Contactologia. 1993;15E: 177–189.

Bialasiewicz A, Janssen K. Inflammatory disorders of the outer eye and anterior segment—classification, differential diagnosis, microbiology—part 2: episcleritis, scleritis, keratitis, trabeculitis. Contactologia. 1994;16E: 34–42.

Bieri F. A device for examining contact lenses at the slit lamp. Contactologia. 1989;11E: 191–193.

van Bijsterveld OP, Klaassen-Broekema N. Contact lenses and pseudomonas infection. Contactologia. 1994;16E: 66–68.

Bonnet M. Epsilon aminocaproic acid and tear film. Contactologia. 1991;13E: 12–13.

Boy-Miclea M, Cochet P. Radial keratotomy and keratoconus. Contactologia. 1994;16E: 101–116.

Brennan NA, Efron N, Garney LG. Critical oxygen requirements to avoid oedema of the central and peripheral cornea. Acta Ophthalmol. 1987;65: 556–564.

Brethfeld V. Rigid contact lenses: a list of lenses available in the federal republic of Germany in 1989. Contactologia. 1989; 11E: 105–107.

Brethfeld V. Soft contact lenses: a list of lenses available in the federal republic of Germany in 1989. Contactologia. 1989; 11E: 155–158.

Brethfeld V. Rigid contact lenses: a list of lenses available in the federal republic of Germany in 1990. Contactologia. 1990; 12E: 99–101.

Brethfeld V. Soft contact lenses: a list of lenses available in the federal republic of Germany in 1990. Contactologia. 1990; 12E: 145–149

Brethfeld V. Rigid contact lenses: a list of lenses available in the federal republic of Germany in 1991. Contactologia. 1991; 13E: 99–101.

Brethfeld V, Heitz R. Soft contact lenses: a list of lenses available in the federal republic of Germany in 1991. Contactologia. 1991;13E: 147–151.

Brewitt H. The surface of the eye in health and disease—selected problems in contactology. Contactologia. 1991;13E: 1–7.

Brewitt H. Clinical study on the compatibility and efficacy of Proxcid enzyme cleaner and the Proxcid disinfecting system. Contactologia. 1992;14E: 166–174.

Brewitt H, Mandel S. Contact lens care systems: alphabetical list of cleaning, disinfection and storage solutions available in the federal republic of Germany. Contactologia. 1989;11E: 53–58.

Brewitt H, Mandel S. Contact lens care systems: alphabetical list of cleaning, desinfection and storage solutions available in the federal republic of Germany. Contactologia. 1990;12E: 1–8.

Brewitt H, Mandel S. Contact lens care system: alphabetical list of cleaning, disinfection and storage solutions available in the federal republic of Germany. Contactologia. 1991;13E: 49–54.

Brewitt H, Mandel S. Contact lens care systems: alphabetical list of cleaning, disinfection and storage solutions available in the Federal Republic of Germany. Contactologia. 1992;14E: 1–8.

Brewitt H, Driller H, Török M. Comparison of Thilo – tears Gel and Methocel Dispersa in diagnostic contact lens examination of the eye. Contactologia. 1994;16E: 117–126.

Brewitt H, Beushausen D, Joost P, Riesmeier M, Sander U, Wildner B. Rewetting of contact lenses: clinical data on efficacy and indications. Contactologia. 1994;16E: 87–95.

Bruce AS, Brennan NA. Corneal pathophysiology with contact lens wear. Surv opthalmol. 1990;35: 25–58.

Bürki E. Materials for hard and soft contact lenses. Contactologia. 1989;11E: 1–4.

Bürki E. Office modification of rigid lenses. Contactologia. 1989;11E: 34–44.

Bürki E. Systematic fitting of rigid and soft contact lenses using the sagittal radii measuring method part 1: theoretical principles. Contactologia. 1989;11E: 63–73.

Bürki E. The systematic fitting of rigid and soft contact lenses using the sagittal radii method—part 2: practical results. Contactologia. 1990;12E: 72–76.

Bürki E. Corneal topography—comparison between manual evaluation and the automatic KR 3500 kerato/refractometer. Contactologia. 1992;14E: 129–132.

Bürki E. Fluorescein photography in contact lens practice. Contactologia. 1992;14E: 162–165

Bürki E. Videokeratometry and contact lens fitting. Contactologia. 1995;17E: 68–76.

Campello Lloret J. Correction of astigmatism with contact lenses: a study of five types of toric soft lenses. Contactologia. 1992;14E: 9–13.

Capoferri C, Sirianni P, Menga M. Pseudomonas keratitis in disposable soft lens wear. Contactologia. 1991;13E: 61–62.

Cavanagh HD. Use of therapeutic hydrogel in corneal melting disorders. Contactologia. 1995;17E: 177–181.

Claas W. Systematic fitting of contact lenses. Contactologia. 1993;15E: 18–25.

Claas W, Kohlmann H, Lommatzsch PK, Busse H. Studies of contact lens deposits using fluorescein-conjugated antibodies and antibody-labelled magnetic particles. Contactologia. 1991;13E: 30–34.

Cochet P, Armiad H. The shape of the cornea. Contactologia. 1995;17E: 33–40.

Cochet P, Dezard X. Pseudokeratoconus and its relevance to contact lens wear. Contactologia. 1994;16E: 153–158.

Cochet P, Dezard X, Caillaud S. Videokeratographic documentation of keratoconus. Contactologia. 1994;16E: 19–25.

Colin J, Malet F, Robinet A, Heitz R. The epidemiology of acanthamoeba keratitis in Europe. Contactologia. 1990;12E: 54–56.

Colin J, Malet F, Richard MC, Chastel C. Collagen shields in the treatment of herpes simplex keratitis. Contactologia. 1991;13E: 23–25.

Coursaux G. Visual comfort of central near vision contact lenses to correct presbyopia—theoretical considerations. Contactologia. 1989;11E: 120–121.

Coursaux G, Corbe C, Saraux H. Correction of presbyopia with "super-zoom" lenses: clinical and physiological studies. Contactologia. 1989;11E: 122–125.

Coursaux G, Bloch-Michel E, Fellous JC, Massin M. Refitting of gigant papillary conjunctivitis patients with Acuvue disposable contact lenses. Contactologia. 1990;2E : 26–28.

Dabezies OH, Cavanagh HD, Farris RL, Lemp MA. Contact lenses. The CLAO guide to basic science and clinical practice. Orlando:Grune and Stratton;1984.

Damms T, Hadjian R, Winter R. Chemofluorescence with calcofluor white for the detection of acanthamoeba in patients with keratitis: a retrospective study on 152 corneal buttons after keratoplasty. Contactologia. 1994;16E : 159–165.

Dannheim F, Stiller H. Influence of spectacles or contact lenses on the visual field. Contactologia. 1994;16E : 173–177.

de Decker W. Relationship between the development of visual functions in children and correction of ametropia. Contactologia. 1995;17E : 15–21.

Dezard X, Caillaud S, Cochet P. Biometric casts for fitting contact lenses in keratoconus. Contactologia. 1992;14E : 155–161.

Dezard X, Caillaud S, Cochet P. Indications for soft bandage lenses in corneal dystrophies and corneal degenerations. Contactologia. 1994;16E : 133–137.

Diamond JP, Dallas NL, Warr R. Fitting irregular corneal grafts with contact lenses. Contactologia. 1992;14E : 143–145.

Donshik PC, Ballow M. Tear immunoglobulins in giant papillary conjunctivitis induced by contact lenses. Am J Ophthalmol. 1983;96 : 460–466.

Donshik PC, Luistro AE. Hybrid gas permeable – soft contact lens. Contactologia. 1990;12E : 32–34.

Donshik PC, Luistro AE. A comparison of three new soft bifocal contact lenses. Contactologia. 1991;13 E;39–41.

Doughman DJ. Contact lens uses as a therapeutic tool—unstable epithelium, recurrent erosion, bullous keratopathy and filamentary keratitis. Contactologia. 1995;17E : 182–188.

Dreifus M, Schimmelpfennig B. The thermal properties of the rabbit cornea in contact lens wear. Contactologia. 1990; 12E : 60–62.

Drobec P. Rigid contact lens migration through upper lid tissue. Contactologia. 1994;16E : 127–128.

Eder-Schmid R. Successful treatment of suspected acanthamoeba keratitis associated with soft lens wear. Contactologia. 1994;16E : 59–60.

Efron N, Morgan PB. Hydrogel contact lens dehydration and oxygen transmissibility. CLAO J. 1999;25 : 148–151.

Eggink FAGJ, Beekhuis WH. Contact lens fitting following radial keratotomy and other relaxing incisions. Contactologia. 1989;11E : 164–168.

Eggink FAGJ, Pinckers AJL, Aandekerk AL. Subepithelial opacities in daily wear high water content soft contact lenses. Contactologia. 1991;13E : 173–176.

Eggink FAGJ, Pinckers AJLG, Graaf de R. Two soft concentric varifocal contact lenses. Contactologia. 1993;15E : 26–29.

Ehrich W. The aetiology of limbal hyperaemia and vascularization caused by HEMA lenses. Contactologia. 1989;11E : 188–190.

Ehrich W. Prevention of acanthamoeba keratitis. Contactologia. 1991;13E : 26–28.

Ehrich W. The first fifty years of contact lenses: measurement of corneal and scleral curvature. Contactologia. 1991;13E : 69–80.

Ehrich W. History of contact lenses—the first fifty years protective shells, bandage lenses, lenses for albinism and drug delivery. Contactologia. 1992;14E : 90–95.

Ehrich W. The first fifty years of contact lenses: diagnostic shells and the hydrodiascope. Contactologia. 1994;16E : 2–6.

Ehrich W. The first fifty years of contact lenses: keratoconus. Contactologia. 1994;16E : 7–12.

Ehrich W, Epstein D. Color Atlas of Contact Lenses. Stuttgart:Thieme;1988.

Ehrich W, Höh H. The anterior chamber test of plastics—number of animals required and evaluation methods. Contactologia. 1989;11E : 130–137.

Elcioglu M, Kir N, Gezer A, Közer Bilgin L, Akarcay K. Interference studies of the tear film lipid layer. Contactologia. 1990; 12E : 35–38.

Elie G. Continuous wear of contact lenses—rigid gas permeability or disposable lenses? Contactologia. 1992;14E : 185–188.

Elie G. Contamination of contact lens solutions. Contactologia. 1995;17E : 93–97.

Esgin H, Erda N. Endothelial cell density of the cornea during rigid gas permeable contact lens wear. CLAO J. 2000;26 : 204–213.

Fanti P. Results of high water content lens wear over a period of seven years. Contactologia. 1990;12E : 121–126.

Fatt I, Freeman RD, Lin D. Oxygen tension distribution in the Cornea. Exp. Eye res. 1974;18 : 357–365.

Fernandez del Cotero Munoz JN, Velarde Rodriguez JJ, Vega de la Torre F. The corneal endothelium and contact lens wear. Contactologia. 1993;15E : 157–162.

Fourny A. Clinical study of a new rigid gas-permeable elliptic lens: evaluation of 251 eyes. Contactologia. 1989;11E : 74–76.

Fourny A, Kantelip B, Amrouche M. Scanning electron microscopic observations of the anterior surface of unused gas-permeable rigid lenses. Contactologia. 1989;11E : 77–80.

Fourny A, Kantelip B, Amrouche M. Scanning electron microscopic study of the front surface of rigid gas permeable lenses: daily and extended wear contact lenses. Contactologia. 1989;11E : 159–163.

Freeman MI, Hovander CR. Experiences with a rigid gas permeable tangential segment bifocal contact lens. Contactologia. 1991;13E : 90–92.

Fritsch R. Daily wear of disposable lenses with frequent lens replacement. Contactologia. 1992;14 : 77–83.

Fuhr B. Ciprofloxacin as a topical antimicrobial drug. Contactologia. 1995;17E : 146–153.

Fukazawa A, Kanai A, Itoi M, Kobuci T, Itagai T. Corneal endothelium change due to wearing disposable soft contact lenses. J Jpn Cl Soc. 2002;44 : 172–175.

Fushimi N. Wound healing of corneal epithelium. J Jpn Cl Soc. 2001;43 : 183–196.

Gabriels GJH, Emmerich KH, Busse H, Conrads H. Radial keratotomy: an experimental study in rabbits. Contactologia. 1990;12E : 63–70.

Garcia Gómez S, Bairreiro Rego A, Garcia Delpech S. Fluorescein and corneal epithelialization: an experimental study. Contactologia. 1991;13E : 123–127.

Garcia Gómez S, Barreiro Rego A, Garcia Delpech S. Corneal thickness in rabbit eyes—lid closure vs. bandage lenses. Contactologia. 1992;14E : 23–27.

Garcia Gómez S, Garcia Delpech S, Garcia Delpech E. Collagen shields in cataract surgery. Contactologia. 1993;15E : 59–63.

Garrigue G, Brémont S, Burguie're AM, Poveda JD. Bactericidal activity of six contact lens care solutions—a comparative study. Contactologia. 1995;17E : 1–10.

Gernet H. Oculometric findings in myopia. Doc. Ophthalmol. 1981;28 : 71–77.

Geyer OC. Anduran, a successful material for contact lenses. Contactologia. 1989;11E : 31–33.

Geyer OC, Wagenbach G, Böhme A. Scleral lenses today—applications and manufacturing methods. Contactologia. 1995;17E : 168–176.

Gioia de E, Musso M, Ligorio MC, Perino P, Bove MS, Grignolo FM. Treatment of amblyopia with contact lenses. Contactologia. 1995;17E : 88–92.

Göbbels M, Ohlhorst D, Spitznas M. Endothelial permeability in long—term contact lens wearers with deep stromal opacities—a prospective fluorophotometric study. Contactologia. 1991;13E : 18–22.

Goede GH. Is rigid contact lens adherence due to hydromechanical causes? Contactologia. 1991;13E : 114–122.

Gottesleben I. Presbyopia in contact lens practice. Contactologia. 1991;13E : 106–109.

Gubert N. "Variations", a new contact lens for presbyopic patients. Contactologia. 1991;13E : 110–111.

Güler C, Bakici Z, Yüksel N, Caglar Y. Bacterial contamination of soft contact lens solutions. Contactologia. 1990;12E : 106–109.

Guillon M, Guillon JP, Shah D, Williams J. Visual performance stability of planned replacement daily wear contact lenses. Contactologia. 1995;17E:118–130.

van Haeringen NJ. Inhibition of lysozyme activity by preservatives. Contactologia. 1993;15E:68–71.

Hagenah M, Insler MS, Hill JM. Minimal hydration required for optimal absorbition of epidermal growth factor into a corneal shield. Contactologia. 1994;16E:149–152.

Hagenah M, Lopez JG, Insler MS. Effects of EGF, acidic FGF, and collagen shields on epithelial wound healing in rabbits following superficial keratectomy. Contactologia. 1994;16E:143–148.

Hansen FK. A clinical study of the normal human central corneal thickness. Acta Ophthalmol. 1971;49:82–89.

Hara Y, Miyamoto K. Immunoreactions in the eye. J Jpn Cl Soc. 2001;43:126–132.

Hartstein J. Corneal warping due to the wearing of contact lenses. Am J Opthalmol. 1965;60:1103–1104.

Hartstein J. The joys and dangers of contact lenses. New York:Carlton Press;1988.

Heffinck P. Computerized assisted choice of first rigid trial lens in cases of high astigmatismus. Contactologia. 1990;12E:150–154.

Heister H, Heller K. A new rigid gas permeable lens (Quantum). Contactologia. 1989;11E:126–129.

Heitz R, Gast E, Floesser R, Hauth JC. Two cases of pseudomonas keratitis in soft contact lens wearers. Contactologia. 1989;11E:96–101.

Herde J. Keratitis in a monocular aphakic diabetic fitted with an extended wear lens. Contactologia. 1994;16E:61–65.

Herde J. Wilhelms D, Paschold S, Tost M. Conjunctival flora af soft lens wearers, spectacle wearers and emmetropes in a polluted environment. Contactologia. 1991;13E:134–136.

Höh H. Correction of unilateral myopia with contact lenses. Contactologia. 1991;13E:156–168.

Höh H. Bandage lenses, bandage shells and contact shells. Contactologia. 1993;15E:83–94.

Höh H, Behr M. Refractive changes following Nd: YAG laser keratotomy—importance of laser parameters. Contactologia. 1990;12E:22–25.

Höh H, Ruprecht KW. The use of contact lenses in metabolic diseases. Contactologia. 1994;16E:69–73.

Höh H, Kienecker C, Ruprecht KW. Correction of unilateral refractive errors with contact lenses in infancy and early childhood. Contactologia. 1993;15E:105–115.

Höh H, Schirra F, Kienecker C, Ruprecht KW. Lid-parallel conjunctival fold (LIPCOF) and dry eye: a diagnostic tool for the contactologist. Contactologia. 1995;17E:104–117.

Hoevding G. A clinical study of the association between thickness and curvature of the central cornea. Acta Ophthalmol.1983;61:461–466.

Holden B. Corneal swelling response to contact lens worn under extended wear conditions. Invest Ophthalmol Vis Sci. 1983;24:218–226.

Holden B. A report card on hydrogen peroxide for contact lens disinfection. CLAO J. 1990;16:61–64.

Holden B, Sweeny DF, Efron N, Vannas A, Nilson KT. Contact lenses can induce stromal thinning. Clin exp Optom. 1988;71:109–113.

Holly F. The preocular tear film. Lubbock:Dry eye institute;1986.

Houttequiet I, Derous D, Dieltiens M, Missoten L. The influence of contact lenses on corneal curvature. Contactologia. 1986;8E:53–56.

Ichijma H, Hayashi T, Mitsunaga S, Hamano H. Determination of oxygen tension on rabbits cornea under contact lenses. CLAO J.1998;24:220–226.

Itoi M, Kanai A. The Necessety of a regular follow-up examination in disposable soft contact lens wearers. J Jpn CL Soc. 2001;43:142–154.

Iwasaki W, Takayama M, Kosaka Y, Roth HW. Clinical trials, using an elliptical lens. J Jpn CL Soc. 1982;34:310–315.

Jahn D. Pseudochalazion due to a "lost" contact lens. Contactologia. 1992;14E:96–97.

Janoff L, Dabezies OH. Power change induced by soft contact lens flexure. CLAO J. 1983;9:32–38.

Junker FK. The importance of sagittal height and of total diameter in fitting contact lenses. Contactologia. 1989;11E:112–119.

Kaiser L. Preservative-free ophthalmic drugs. Contactologia. 1992;14E:49–52.

Kanpolat A, Yilmaz M, Batioglu F, Akbas F. Piggyback contact lenses revisited. Contactologia. 1994;16E:129–132.

Kasperski S. Advantages and disposable lenses of etafilcon disposable leses. Contactologia. 1992;14E:74–76.

Kaufman H, Barron B, McDonald M, Waltman S. The Cornea. New York:Livingstone,1988.

Kemmetmüller H. Critical thoughts about the transformation of the corneal curvature by wearing contact lenses. Contact. lens J. 1983;11:3–11.

Kersley HJ. Extended or daily wear—is disposability the way? Contactologia. 1989;11E:108–111.

Key JE. Hydron Echelon diffractive soft bifocal lens for presbyopia. Contactologia. 1990;12E:89–92.

Key JE, Yee JL. Prospective clinical evaluation of the Acuvue bifocal contact lens. CLAO J. 1999;25:218–221.

Knop E, Brewitt H. Clinical studies on Weflex 55 and the Polyrinse cleaning and disinfection system. Contactologia. 1989;11E:22–26.

Knop E, Brewitt H. Morphology of the conjunctival epithelium in spectacle and contact lens wearers—a light and elektron microscopic study. Contactologia. 1992;14E:108–120.

Koetting RA, Castellano CF, Keating MJ. PMMA lenses worn for twenty years. J Am Optom Ass. 1986;57:459–461.

Kohlhaas M, Lerche RC, Draeger J. Lamellar corneal dissection techniques: the state of the art. Contactologia. 1995;17E:131–138.

Kohm TH, Draeger J. Correlation of changes in corneal sensitivity to lens power in contact lens wearers. Contactologia. 1993;15E:124–130.

Kok JHC, Vreugdenhil W. Extended wear of high oxygen permeability Boston Equa and Fluoroperm contact lenses. Contactologia. 1990;12E:163–167.

Kranning HJ, Ehrich W. H_2O_2 stress of contact lenses. Contactologia. 1989;11E:176–187.

Krause A. Intracorneal biocompatibility of glass ceramics. Contactologia. 1992;14E:28–31.

Kreiss-Gosselin F. Correction of ametropia with contact lenses. Contactologia. 1995;17E:142–145.

Kreis-Gosselin F, Lumbroso P. Extended wear of rigid gas permeable, high Dk contact lenses in myopia. Contactologia. 1990;12E:158–162.

Kuckelkorn R, Reim M. The contact lens as "artificial epithelium" in eye burns. Contactologia. 1994;16E:74–81

Lagoutte F. Prevention of acanthamoeba keratitis in contact lens weares. Contactologia. 1994;16E:49–53.

Laroche G. Case report: undetected glaucoma in a long-term contact lens wearer. Contactologia. 1990;12E:93–95.

Lebow KA, Grohe RM. Differentiating contact lens induced warpage from true keratoconus using corneal topography. CLAO J. 1999;25:114–122.

Lee AM, Kastl PR. Rigid gas permeable contact lens fitting after radial keratomy. CLAO J. 1998;24:33–35.

Leluan P, Liotet S, Batellier L, Chaumeil C. Amoebic and bacterial contamination of contact lens storage cases—a study of 32 keratitis patients and 63 healthy lens wearers. Contactologia. 1991;13E:137–141.

Lemp MA, Marquardt R. The dry eye. Berlin:Springer;1992.

Liesegang TJ. Contact lens related conjunctivitis. Cornea. 1997;16:265–273.

Lin A, Driebe WT, Polack P. Alcaligenes xylosoxidans keratitis post penetrating keratoplasty in a rigid gas-permeable wearer. CLAO J. 1998;24:239–241.

Liotet S, Rault J. Scanning electron microscopic study of contaminated lens storage cases. Contactologia. 1992;14E:63–67.

Liotet S, Sanchez V, Pochet P. Transmissibility of antibiotics in 38% and 70% water content hydrophilic soft lenses. Contactologia. 1993;15E : 163–166.

Liotet S, Xerri B, Batellier L, Chaumeil C. Pitfalls in contact lens disinfection. Contactologia. 1989;11E : 141–147.

Liotet S, Xerri B, Chaumeil C, Batellier L. Analysis of proteins in tear protein anomalies. Contactologia. 1989;11E : 138–140.

Liotet S, Vassor A, Benchetrit D, Chaumeil C, Batellier L, Xerri B. Influence of material on the adherence of bacteria to contact lenses. Contactologia. 1990;12E : 47–53.

Lipener C, Ribeiro ALP. Bilateral pseudomonas ulceration in disposable contact lens wearer. CLAO J. 1999;25 : 123–124.

López Alemany A, Presencia Redal A. Giant papillary conjunctivitis in soft and rigid lens wear. Contactologia. 1991;13E : 14–17.

López Alemany A, Campello Lloret J. Evaluation of the effectiveness of peroxide solutions. Contactologia. 1991;13E : 177–182.

López Alemany A, Calleja M, Claramonte P. Effect of non-oxidizing contact lens disinfection system on acanthamoeba culbertsoni. Contactologia. 1992;14E : 68–73.

Lumbroso P, Serpin G, Allard JM. Correction of presbyopia by means of controlled induced myopic anisometropia. Contactologia. 1989;11E : 20–21.

Lumbroso P, Rocher P, Serpin G. Correction of prespyopia—monovision today. Contactologia. 1992;14E : 39–44.

MacKeen DL, Roth HW. Revolutionary method of ocular dry delivery. Invest Ophthalmol Vis Sci. 1995;36 : 166.

MacKeen DL, Roth HW. A simple method of detecting the anti-inflamatory action of topical dry eye treatments. In Sullivan DA: Lacrimal gland, tears film and dry eye syndrome 3. New York: Kluwer Academic;2002.

Maeda N. Disinfection of soft contact lenses. J Jpn Cl Soc.2001;43 : 2–10.

Maeyens E, Houttequiet I, Misotten L. Corneal grafts and contact lens fitting. Contactologia. 1994;16E : 96–100.

Malet F. Correction of low myopia: disposable lenses or radial keratotomy? Contactologia. 1992;14E : 14–16.

Maréchal-Courtois CH, Vanhakendover C, Delcourt JC. Clincial evaluation of the opti-free disinfecting system with european hydrophilic contact lenses. Contactologia. 1992;14E : 181–184.

Maréchal-Courtois CH, Duchesne B, Delcourt JC, Feiss L. Fitting contact lenses in patients with corneal grafts. Contactologia. 1993;15E : 72–75.

Marquardt R. Tear film stability and the immune barrier. Contactologia. 1993;15E : 174–176.

Marquardt R, König C. Soluble inserts for the treatment of dry eye. Contactologia. 1991;13E : 183–188.

Marquardt R, Roth HW, Laux U. Experiments with a new large diameter soft contact lens. Contact Lens J. 1975;3 : 9–19.

Martola EL, Baum JL. Central and peripheral corneal thickness. Arch Ophthalmol. 1968;79 : 28–30.

Mathers WD. Therapeutic contact lenses in eyelid and conjunctival disease. Contactologia. 1995;17E : 189–192.

Mathers WD. Why the cornea becomes dry? CLAO J. 2000;26 : 159–165.

Mawas LJ, Fateh S. Strabismus and disposable contact lenses. Contactologia. 1995;17E : 139–141.

Mayer W, Ulmer W, Schmidauer CH. Ptosis and contact lenses. Contactologia. 1992;14E : 36–38.

Mestres P. Shape and attachment of L-929 cells cultured on contact lenses. Contactologia. 1994;16E : 26–33.

Michielsen B, Kempeneers A, Houttequiet I, Missotten L. Disposable soft contact lenses. Contactologia. 1990;12E : 178–180.

Miller B. Keratoconus—new contact lens geometries for steep cones. Contactologia. 1990;12E : 7–12.

Miller B. Bifocal contact lenses: optical principles. Contactologia. 1992;14E : 98–100.

Miller B. Toric contact lenses for high astigmatism, aspheric and asymmetrically decentred lenses for advanced keratoconus. Contactologia. 1994;16E : 13–18.

Millis E. Corneal complications of extended soft lens wear in diabetics. Contactologia. 1993;15E : 35–40.

Missiroli A, Mancino R, Pocobelli A, Ricci F, Cerulli L. In vitro evaluation of serum complement changes induced by contact lenses. Contactologia. 1992;14E : 125–128.

Mizutani Y, Yoshinori S. The effect of CO_2 on the cornea. J Jpn Cl Soc. 1991;3 : 234–241.

MönksT, Busin M. Computerized corneal topography. Contactologa. 1993,15E : 167–173.

Monestier-Carlus D, Cochet P. Case report: 23 years of PMM extended wear. Contactologia. 1989;11E : 148–149.

Montard M, Bosc JM. Intraocular lens implantation or keratomileusis? Results of refractive surgery in high myopia. Contactologia. 1990;12E : 130–138.

Morgan JF. Factors in compliance: contact lens hygiene. Contactologia. 1993,15E : 116–123.

Morgan PB, Efron N. Hydrogel contact lens ageing. CLAO J. 2000;26 : 91–96.

Müller-Lierheim WGK. European standards and the EG medical devices directive. Contactologia. 1993;15E : 10–17.

Murube del Castillo J. Dacryologia Basica. Madrid:Royper;1982.

Nicaise P, Liotet S, Batellier L, Chaumeil C. The importance of quantitative analysis of various fractions when interpreting the electrophoresis of tear proteins. Contactologia. 1989;11E : 81–83.

Nilsson SEG, Lindh H. Disposable contact lenses—a prospective study of clinical performance in flexible and extended wear. Contactologia. 1990;12E : 80–88.

Nilsson SEG, Lindh H. Polyquad and hydrogen peroxide disinfecting solutions—a comparison of subjective comfort and objective findings. Contactologia. 1990;12E : 102–105.

Nilsson SEG, Söderquist M. Monovision with disposable contact lenses, a six-month prospective study. Contactologia. 1992; 14E : 53–61.

Nossin F, Houttequiet I, Missotten L. Bandage contact lenses—indications and results. Contactologia. 1995;17E : 41–44.

Odenthal MTHP, Eggink FAGJ, Vreugdenhil W, Beekhuis WH. Corneal response to Quantum II rigid gas permeable extended wear lenses. Contactologia. 1993;15E : 30–34.

Ohya S, Takahashi K, Murakami A, Nakayasu K. Complications in soft lens wearers. J Jpn Cl Soc. 2001;43 : 97–102.

Opel H, Ris W. The tear film and its interference patterns. Contactologia. 1990;12E : 181–186.

Opel H, Ris W. Fluorocon PE, an alternative to soft contact lenses. Contactologia. 1992;14E : 84–89.

Or KH, Erda N, Gönenc D. Complications in the use of contact lenses in aphakia. Contactologia. 1990;12E : 118–120.

Osuský R. A method for rapidly estimating corneal eccentricity. Contactologia. 1990;12E : 77–79.

Pace PH, Dufier J. Comparative study of soft diffractive lenses and the monovision system. Contactologia. 1992;14E : 137–140.

Pace P, Guyot-Sionet P, Vidal R, Giorgi G, Jonard M. A new concept in contactology: disposable lenses. Contactologia. 1989; 11E : 59–62.

Pace PH, Liotet S. Bacteriological study of disposable contact lenses worn for 1–2 weeks. Contactologia. 1990;12E : 171–172.

Pelzer I, Raab U. Steroid-antibiotic combination therapy. Contactologia. 1995;17E : 193–197.

Perry HD, Donnenfeld ED, Grossman GA, Stein M, Epstein AB. Retained aspergillus-contaminated contact lens inducing conjunctival mass and keratoconjunctivitis in an immunocompetent patient. CLAO J. 1998;24 : 57–58.

Pescosolido N, Lupelli L, Brosio E, Delfini M, D'Ubaldo A, Verzegnassi B. Nuclear magnetic resonance study of dehydration in a glyceryl-methyl-methacrylate contact lens. Contactologia. 1993;15E : 64–67.

Petroutsos G, Stefanou S, Mavridis A, Psilas K. Acanthamoeba keratitis in a contact lens wearer. The first case in Greece. Contactologia. 1992;14E : 141–144.

Porazinski AD, Donshik PC. Giant papillary conjunctivitis in frequent replacement contact lens wearers: a retrospective study. CLAO J. 1999;25 : 142–147.

Portten M, Brewitt H, Nason RJ. The surface of used disposable contact lenses—a scanning electron microscopy study. Contactologia. 1993;15E : 55–58.

Posenauer B. Rigid contact lenses: a list of lenses available in Germany on 1992. Contactologia. 1992;14E : 105–107.

Polse KA, Rivera RK, Bonnano J. Ocular effects of hard gas-permeable-lens extended wear. Amer J Optom Physiol Opt.1988;65 : 358–364.

Quesnel NM, Simonet P. Efficacy of uv-absorbing contact lenses. Contactologia. 1995;17E : 53–67.

Ratzkova A, Kienecker C, Ruprecht KW. On the progression of Keratoconus. Contactologia. 1995;17E : 11–14.

Rebert H, Koffel JC. Evaluation of thimerosal binding by rigid gas permeable lenses. Contactologia. 1989;11E : 172–175.

Recupero SM, Leucci E, Fasano D, Pacella E, Palma S. Clinical experience with extended wear rigid gas permeable contact lenses. Contactologia. 1991;13E : 128–130.

Ren DH, Matthew P, Jester JV, Ho-fan J, Cavanagh HD. Short term hypoxia downregulates epithelial cell desquamation in vivo but does not increase pseudomonas aeruginosa adherence to exfoliated human corneal epithelial cells. CLAO J. 1999;25 : 73–79.

Ren DH, Matthew P, Jester JV, Ho-fan J, Cavanagh HD. The relationship betwenn contact lens oxygen permeability and binding of pseudomonas aeruginosa to human epithelial cells after overnight and extended wear. CLAO J. 1999;25 : 80–95.

Rengstorff RH. Corneal refraction:relative effects of each corneal component. J Am Optom Ass. 1985;56 : 218–219.

Rengstorff RH, Nilson KT. Long-term effects of extended wear lenses:changes in refraction, corneal curvature, and visual acuity. Am J Optom Physiol Opt.1985;62 : 66–68.

Rolando M, Giordano G, Brezzo V, Murialdo U, Calabria G. Collagen shields to promote epithelial healing in keratoconjunctivitis sicca. Contactologia. 1992;14E : 32–35.

Roth HW. Indications, contraindications and therapeutic use of highwater content soft hydrophilic contact lenses. J Jpn Cl Soc. 1978;21 : 175–179.

Roth HW. Results of a long term study to compare cold sterilization and aseptization of soft hydrophilic contact lenses. Concilium ophthalmol. 1978;23 : 1244–1247.

Roth HW. The etiology of ocular irritation in soft lens wearers:distribution in a large clinical sample. Contact and intraocular lens med. J. 1978;4 : 38–47.

Roth HW. Soft hydrophilic contact lenses. Results of a long term study. J Jpn Cl Soc. 1979;21 : 18–21.

Roth HW. Orthokeratology on children. Experience with the myopia progressiva. The Contact Lens Journal.1980;8 : 6–7.

Roth HW. Dendritic corneal lesions caused by contact lenses. Contactologia. 1990;12E : 115–117.

Roth HW. Disposable lenses: indications and tolerance. Contactologia. 1990;12E : 173–177.

Roth HW. The etiology and pathogenesis of corneal ulcers in contact lens wearers. Contactologia. 1990;12E : 110–114.

Roth HW. Polyquad-induced mixed solution syndrome in contact lens wear. Contactologia. 1991;13E : 8–11.

Roth HW. Studies on the etiology and treatment of giant papillary conjunctivitis in contact lens wearers. Contactologia. 1991;13E : 55–60.

Roth HW. The causes of contact lens loss. Contactologia. 1991;13E : 35–38.

Roth HW. Differentiation of keratoconus types by micropachymetry. Contactologia. 1992;14E : 17–22.

Roth HW. Corneal scarring after long-term rigid contact lens wear. Contactologia. 1993;15E : 138–142.

Roth HW. Micropachometric investigation of rigid contact lens-induced corneal dystrophies. CLAO J. 1993;2 : 129–132.

Roth HW. Problems of Contact Lens Hygiene. Arab Medico. 1993;6 : 17–19.

Roth HW. A new piggyback contact lens system for presbyopia. Contactologia. 1995;17E : 162–167.

Roth HW. New syndrome identified in daily contact lens wear. Optometry Today. 1998;7 : 7–19.

Roth. HW, Roth-Wittig M. Contact-Lenses. A Handbook for Patients. Hagerstone:Harper and Row;1980.

Roth HW, Roth-Wittig M. Multipurpose solutions for soft lens maintenance. International Contact Lens Clinic. 1980; 17 : 13–16.

Roth HW, Iwasaki W, Takayama M, Wada C. Complication caused by Silicon Elastomer Lenses. Contacto. 1980;24 : 28–36.

Roth-Wittig M, Roth HW. The use of multipurpose solutions for soft lens maintenance. The Contact Lens J. 1980;9 : 34–36.

Rowsey JJ, Reynolds AE, Brown R. Corneal topography. Arch. Ophthalmol. 1981;99 : 1073–1100.

Ruben M. Contact Lens Practice. London:Tindall;1975.

Ruben M, Lena W, Chu F. Radial keratotomy transmission electron microscopic studies on the rabbit. Contactologia. 1989;11E : 5–14.

Schanzlin DJ, Robin BJ. Corneal Topography. Heidelberg:Springer;1991.

Schmidt HHJ, Diekstall FF, Manns MP. Corneal opacities in patients with complete or partial lecithin-cholesterol acyltransferase deficiency: lCAT deficiency and fish-eye disease. Contactologia. 1995;17E : 77–80.

Schmidt M, Döring C, Wegner A. The therapeutic effect of collagen shields. Contactologia. 1994;16E : 54–58.

Schmidt M, Merté RL, Torster A, Mertz M. Contact lens fitting in infants. Contactologia. 1995;17E : 22–27.

Schneider G. Legal issues in contact lens practice. Contactologia. 1995;17E : 28–32.

Schoessler JP. Corneal endothelial polymegathism assiciated with extended wear. Int contact lens clinic. 1983;10 : 148–155.

Schunk R, Schweisfurth R. Disinfectant performance of oxidizing contact lens solutions: quantitative suspension tests with organic contaminants. Contactologia. 1989;11E : 84–89.

Schunk T, Schweisfurth R. Disinfectant performance of oxidizing care system on organically contaminated contact lenses. Contactologia. 1989;11E : 90–95.

Sengör T, Gürgül S, Ögretmenoglu S, Kilic A, Erker H. Tear immunology in contact lens wearers. Contactologia. 1990;12E : 43–45.

Seyfarth M, Janietz U. Investigation of secretory Iga in the lacrimal fluid. Contactologia. 1991;13E : 152–154.

Shaw EL. Practical uses of collagen lenses. Contactologia. 1990; 12E : 29–31.

Silva V, Santos Ferreira R, Andrade L, et al. Complications of aphakic extended wear rigid gas permeable contact lenses. Contactologia. 1991;13E : 131–133.

Spraul CW, Roth, HJG, Gäckle H, Lang GE, Lang KL. Influence of special effect contact lenses (crazy lenses) on visual function. CLAO J. 1998;24 : 29–32.

Stapleton F, Lakshmi KR, Sweeny DF, Rao GN, Holden BA. Overnight swelling in symptomatic and asymptomatic contact lens wearers. CLAO J. 1998;24 : 169–174.

Stein HA, Slatt BJ, Stein RM. Fitting guide for rigid and soft contact lenses: A practical approach. St. Louis:Mosby,1990.

Stein H, Caffery B, Fontana F, et al. Clinical evaluation of a new polyquad—preserved rigid gas permeable contact lens system. Contactologia. 1995;17E : 45–48

Stern GA. Contact lens associated bacterial keratitis: past, present, future. CLAO J. 1998;24 : 52–56.

Stevenson R, Vaja N, Jackson J. Corneal transparency chances resulting from osmotic stress. Ophthalm Opt.1983;3 : 33–39.

Stolze HH, Becker J. Corneal responses to UV-induced free radicals. Contactologia. 1993;15E : 143–145.

Sucheki JK, Ehlers WH, Donshik PC. A comparision of contact lens-related complications in various daily wear modalities. CLAO J. 2000;26 : 215–218.

Szymankiewicz S, Roth HW, Szymankiewicz M. Soctewski kontaktowe w practyce okulistycznej oraz powiklania. Warsawa:Oftal;2001.

Temel A, Kazokoglu H, Taga Y. The effect of contact lens wear on tear immunoglobulins. Contactologia. 1990;12E : 39–42.

Tervo T, Virtanen T, Setten van GB. The proteolitic system and contact lens wear. Contactologia. 1993;15E : 76–82.

Thill-Schwaninger M. Recognition of random dot stereograms with blurring or enlargement of one image. Contactologia. 1989;11E:15–19.

Thoft RA, Friend J. Biochemical aspects of contact lens wear. Am J Ophthalmol. 1975;80:139–145.

Tomlinson A. Complications of contact lens wear. St. Louis:Mosby;1992.

Tost F. Conjunctival impression cytology with monoclonal antibodies. Contactologia. 1992;14E:121–124.

Tritten JJ, Tritten-Arber ML, Geinoz J. Bacteriological study of contact lens solutions obtained from keratitis patients. Contactologia. 1990;12E:57–69.

Udell JJ, Meisler DM. Giant papillary conjunctivitis. Int Ophthalm Clin. 1989;26:35–42.

Velasco J, Bermúdez FJ, Ruiz C, Jimenez L, Rubinó M, Hita E. Tear lysozyme activity in wearers of contact lenses. Contactologia. 1995;17E:158–161.

Ververs B, Beekhuis WH, Vreugdenhil W, Eggink FAGJ. The disposable Acuvue contact lens—a pilot study in the Netherlands. Contactologia. 1989;11E:169–171.

Vihlen FS, Wilson G. The relation between eyelid tension, corneal toricity and age. Invest Ophthalmol Vis Sci. 1984;24:1367–1373.

Vogt U. Soft contact lenses—a list of lenses available in the United Kingdom. Contactologia. 1992;14E:149–154.

Vogt U. Contact lens care systems: alphabetical list of cleaning, disinfection and storage solutions available in the united kingdom. Contactologia. 1993;15E:2–9.

Vogt U. Preservative-free ophthalmic drugs. Contactologia. 1993;15E:51–54.

Vogt U. Rigid contact lenses: a list of lenses available in the United Kingdom. Contactologia. 1993;15E:101–104.

Vogt U. Soft contact lenses: a list of lenses available in the United Kingdom. Contactologia. 1993;15E:151–156.

Vreugdenhil W, Eggink FAGJ, Beekhuis WH. Is there an indication for fitting high Dk RGP lenses in former PMMA wearers? Contactologia. 1992;14E:133–136.

Vulpius K, Höh HR, Kienecker CH, Ruprecht KW. Contact lenses in perforating corneal injuries. Contactologia. 1994;16E:166–172.

Weiner S, Mestres P. Morphology of the Detroit 98 epithelial cell line on different contact lens materials (light microscopic findings). Contactologia. 1991;13E:63–67.

Weinstock FJ. The role of disposable contact lenses in presbyopia. Contactologia. 1991;13E:112–113.

Weinstock FJ. Contact Lens Fitting. New York:Lippincott,1998.

Wiederholt M, Broskamp G, Juptner-Johanning D. A clinical study of a new rigid-flexible contact lens with high oxygen transmissibility (Conflex-Air). Contactologia. 1989;11E:27–30.

Wilson AL. External diseases of the eye. Hagerstone:Harper and Row;1979.

Wilson SE, Lin D, Klyce SD, Reidy JJ, Insler MS. Topographic changes in contact lens induced corneal warpage. Ophthalmology. 1990;97:734–737.

Witte T, Brewitt H. Allergic reactions in the conjunctiva and cornea. Contactologia. 1993;15E:131–137.

Ytteborg J, Dohlman C. Corneal edema and intraocular pressure. Arch ophthalmol. 1965;74:477–484.

Zambonin PG, Sabbatini L, Pioggia M, Pocobelli A, Ricci F, Cerulli L. Early detection of protein deposits on soft contact lenses. Contactologia. 1992;14E:175–180.

Index to Text

Acanthamoeba 5, 49, 99, 102, 116
  corneal ulceration 199
AIDS 5, 24, 29, 160
  corneal ulcers 99
albinism 145
allergy 24, 26, 27, 160
  blepharitis 29, 196
  chemosis 42
  complications 190
  conjunctival edema 40
  lens material 86
aniridia 145
antibiotics 198
aphakic patients 6, 78, 125
  babies 24
applanation tonometry 21
Aspergillus 52, 160
astigmatism, irregular 3, 14, 171
automobile accidents 186

bacterial infection 45, 49, 197, 198
beta-blockers 160
binocular vision 21
blepharitis 160
  infectious 29
  squamous 10, 26, 29, 161, 196
blepharoconjunctivitis, allergic 160
blepharospasm 26, 27, 78, 196, 202
blinking 26, 125–6
Bowman's membrane 59, 75, 112
break-up time (BUT) 125, 183
breastfeeding 9

calcium—protein complexes 151
Candida 52, 116, 160
care products 8
cataract 117, 120, 121
chalazion 161
chemical injuries 186, 187, 202
chemotherapy, antineoplastic 5, 24, 160
  corneal ulcers 99
children, follow-up 24
chlorhexidine 88
ciliary injection 54
coagulopathies 160
cobblestone conjunctivitis *see* conjunctivitis, giant papillary
compliance, poor 190, 191
computerized topography 132
conjunctiva 11
  anatomy 35
  bulbar 11, 40
  chemosis 40, 42, 197
  diseases 165, 197–8
  edema 40
  follicular swelling 35
  hemorrhage 42, 197
  hyperemia 11, 45, 52, 80, 198
  injection 52, 78, 102
  irritation 2
  limbus
    injection 54
    neovascularization 14
  mechanical irritation 45
  mixed solution syndrome 88
  necrosis 11

perilimbal injection 54, 80
physiology 35
scarring 27
tarsal 35
trauma 34, 197
conjunctivitis
  acute 165, 176
  bacterial 45, 49, 197, 198
  chronic 165, 171, 173, 176
  fungal 49, 52, 198
  giant papillary 3, 11, 27, 35, 40, 125
    deposits 151
    treatment 197
    wetting problems 138
  Pseudomonas 160
  viral 49, 52, 198
contraindications for contact lenses 4, 9, 10, 190
cornea
  altered curvature 125
  anatomy 59
  bubble formation 75
  clouding 105, 116
  contour changes 110
  cracks 62
  curvature 14
  deformation 200
  diseases 171, 198–200
  edema 60, 75, 80
    glare 127
    glaucoma 117
    impaired vision 125
    improper fitting 123
    tight lens syndrome 78
    treatment 198
    wetting problems 138
  endothelial changes 109
  epithelial changes 59–60, 200
  epithelial defects 66–7, 71, 80, 186
  erosions 66–7, 132, 198
    recurrent 145
  examination 14
  foreign bodies 71
  gas exchange 59
  growths 4
  herpes 24, 71, 171
  hypoxia 66, 75, 115
  indentations 62
  infection 99, 102, 114, 171
  infiltrate 99, 199
  injury 34
  linear grooves 71
  metabolism 3, 114, 173
  mosaics 62, 64
  neovascularization 92, 95, 200
  nummules 64
  oxygen consumption 78
  physiology 59
  pseudoherpetic defects 186, 198
  pseudoinfiltrates 64
  recurrent erosions 171
  scarring 99, 200
  scars 105
  spiders 62
  spiral traces 62
  staining 60

stippling 60
streaks 62, 71
stromal changes 75
swelling 90, 109
  coefficient 114, 115
thickening 75, 78, 109, 112, 127
thickness 60, 114, 184
  central 201
thinning 115
topographical changes 3, 75, 109, 110, 112
topography measurement 123
ulcer 2, 5, 22, 99, 102, 105, 165
  conjunctival trauma 197
  dry eye 176
  keratitis 171
  lens-free interval 195
  prevention 199
  treatment 199
  vascularization 92, 95, 200
corneal deprivation syndrome 90, 199
corneal distortion syndrome 110, 112, 125
cortisone 198, 200
cosmetics 145, 187
counselling of patients 8
cromolyn sodium 197, 199

defective lenses 123
deposits 123, 139, 147, 151
dermatitis, ectopic 26
Descemet's membrane 75, 109, 112
  folds 200
dexpanthenol 198
diabetes mellitus 5, 24, 29, 121
  corneal ulcers 99
  fungal infection 52, 160
discoloration of lenses 145
discontinuation of contact lens wear 195
disinfectant 102
disinfection technique 3, 4, 22, 195
  microbial contamination 99
  thermal 92, 102
disposable lenses 6, 8, 139
  contraindication 90
documentation of findings 23
dry eye 171, 176, 201–2
  syndrome 126, 138
dry-eye ointment 201

ectropion 161
eczema 26
edge defects 139, 186
entropion 161
enzyme tablets 8
examination of patient 10–11
explosives 186
extended-wear lens 78, 80
eye, inner 21, 200
  hypertension 117
  see also intraocular pressure, glaucoma
eye drops 4, 9, 184
  astringent 198, 199
  buffered 67
  corneal anabolic 199
  giant papillary conjunctivitis 197

multivitamin 90
preservative-free 195
thiomersal 40
eye whiteners 198
eyeglass-cleaning solution 187
eyelashes 29, 161
eyelid
abscess 161
anatomy 26
blepharitis 29
disease 161, 196
edema 27, 161, 196
examination 10
infections 29
injury 34, 196
irritation 2, 151
papilloma 161
physiology 26
sebaceous cyst 161
swelling 27
tension 26
trauma 34, 196
ulceration 29

fading of lenses 145
febrile illness 78, 160
fibrin 102, 116
fingernails 130
firecrackers 186
firemen 187
fitting 2, 3, 6, 112, 125
errors 123, 132
poor 114
fluorescein preparations 14
follow-up of wearer 2, 3, 6, 24
foreign bodies 147, 186
cornea 71
frequency of complications 190–1
fungal infection 5, 29, 49, 52, 102, 198
diabetes mellitus 160

gaseous substances 187
gel lenses 14
bandage 198
blepharospasm 26
corneal ulcers 102
gentamicin 199
glare 127, 128, 132, 138
deposits 151
glaucoma 127
tear deficiency 173
glass shards 186
glaucoma 4, 78, 117, 120, 121
fistula 184
glare 127
treatment 200
globe perforation 186
goggle, protective 186
gyrase-inhibitors 198, 199

Haemophilus 49
handling of lens 130, 190
faulty 102, 121
hands of patient 130
hard lenses 8
overwear syndrome 67
PMMA 34
scratches 139
tear deficiency 176
hay fever 160
heparin 197
hepatitis 160

herpes, corneal 24, 71, 171
high risk patients 6
history taking 9
homatropine 199
hormone supplementation 5
hydrogen peroxide 8, 60, 80
chemical injuries 187, 202
cold sterilization 102
hygiene 3, 4, 5, 10, 75, 105, 130
epidemic keratoconjunctivitis 64
inadequate 102
poor 49, 99, 190
hyperopia 78
hypertension 121
intraocular 117
hypopyon 102, 116

immunocompromised patients 5, 29, 34,
92, 105, 116, 160
complications 190
fungal infection 52
see also AIDS; diabetes mellitus; leukemia
infections 5, 9, 10, 22
cornea 99, 102, 114, 171
eyelid 29
ocular 161
see also bacterial infection; conjunctivitis; fungal infection; viral infection
injury risk 6
insertion of lens, faulty 102, 121
inspection
of lens cases 22
of lenses 21
intraocular changes 200
intraocular pressure 21, 78, 80
corneal edema 75
corneal thickness 114
glaucoma 117, 127
toxic keratopathy 86
iridocyclitis 116
iritis 116

Javal ophthalmometer 110
jelly-bump deposits 123, 151

keratitis 171, 176, 197
Acanthamoeba 102
dendritic 71
herpetic 71
metaherpetic 171
Pseudomonas 160
superficial 99
treatment 199
keratitis e lagophthalmo 176
keratoconjunctivitis 86
epidemic 52, 64, 198
keratoconus 6, 64, 109, 125, 171
acute 112
advanced 62
fitting errors 132
Type B 6, 176
Type C 3
keratometer 132
keratopathy
allergic 160
bullous 109, 132, 145, 199
toxic 4, 10, 22, 80, 86
discolored lenses 145
mixed solution syndrome 88
treatment 199

lacrimation
disorders 4, 126, 138, 171
impairment 5, 45, 78
lens care solutions 8, 40, 60, 187, 195
incompatible 88
post-heat syndrome 92
preservative-free 86
lens case 22, 130
lens fragments 130
leukemia 5, 160
corneal ulcers 99
levator dysfunction 196
lissamine green test 183
lodoxamide 197
loss of lenses 4, 121

macular degeneration 117, 121
make-up 145
malignancy 161
malpractice suits 190
manufacture 3
materials 2, 3
defects 139
mechanical injuries 202
medication 5, 9, 145, 160, 190
topical 184
treatment of complications 194
melanoma 165
meniscus test 183
metabolic disease 190
metallic particles 186
microtopography 110
mixed solution syndrome 88
multi-amino acids 199
multivitamins 199
myasthenia gravis 27
mydriasis 21, 116
fixed 145
therapeutic 200
mydriatics 116, 199
myopia 78
corneal pressure 110
high 117, 125
progressive 120

nail polish 145
nandrolone 198
neomycin 199
nevus 165

ocular contusion 186
ocular disease, primary 121, 161
ocular trauma *see* trauma
ophthalmologist
follow-up 2, 6, 24
ocular examination 10
ophthalmometer 132
ophthalmoscopy 117
Ophthalmotest 40, 54, 80, 86
mixed solution syndrome 88
optic neuritis 121
oral contraceptives 5, 9, 151, 160, 190
orthokeratological effects 125
overwear syndrome 66, 67, 132, 195
oxygen, corneal consumption 78
oxygen permeability of lens 59, 102, 132,
200

pachymetry 60, 64, 75, 78, 112
changes 114–15
neovascularization 92
tear deficiency 184

panophthalmitis 99, 116
papillary hypertrophy 35
party lenses 145
pathological conditions 2
patient education 191
pinguecula 4, 165
PMMA lenses 34, 92
    post-heat syndrome 92
Pneumococcus 49
polymyxin B 199
post-heat syndrome 92, 199
pregnancy 9
prescribers 8
preservatives 4, 195
pressure
    chronic 3
    distribution 6
propamidine 199
proptosis 40
pseudoepiscleritis 58
pseudokeratitis bullosa 75
pseudokeratoconus 112
Pseudomonas 5, 49, 99, 102, 116
    conjunctivitis 160
pseudoptosis 27
psychological factors 6
pterygia 4
ptosis 10, 27, 196
punctum lacrimale occlusion 202
punctum plug 202
Pyocyaneus 102

Quincke's edema 27

record keeping 23
refraction changes 121
refractive error 21
renal dysfunction 5
retinal degeneration 145
retinal detachment 117, 120, 121
retinal disease 117
rheumatic disease 5
rigid gas-permeable (RGP) lens 86, 125,
    139, 151
risk factors for complications 190
rose bengal 14, 45
    test 183

salicylate eye baths 196
Sattler's veil 110, 125
Schirmer test 78, 90, 183
Schweitzer mosaic 62
sclera
    anatomy 58
    diseases 198
    hemorrhage 58
    inflammation 58
    injury 34, 58
    pathology 58
    physiology 58
    vasodilatation 58
scopolamine 199
shape of contact lenses 2
silicone lenses 62, 86
silver protein acetyl tannate solution 199
smoking 145
sock phenomenon 151
soft lenses 8
    corneoscleral 34
    fungal infection 52
    hydrophilic 62
    infections 49
    low oxygen permeability 67
    neovascularization 92, 95
    PMMA 92
    silicone 62, 86
    toxic keratopathy 80
spectacle-blur 110, 125
sports 4
Staphylococcus 49
sterilization
    cold 102
    see also disinfection technique
subconjunctival hemorrhage 42
superinfection 29, 198
surface deposits on lenses *see* deposits
systemic disease 5, 160

tear deficiency 78, 161, 171, 173, 201–2
    clinical testing 183
    decompensated 176
    hard lenses 176
tear film abnormality 128
tear flow 26
tear fluid 4, 26, 126, 138

components 151
    pH 78
    refractive index 126, 138
tear lens 126, 138
tear outflow blockage 202
tear-pumping effect 59
tears, artificial 4, 60, 67, 80, 125, 201
thermometry 184
thiomersal 40
    mixed solution syndrome 88
thyroid disease 5
tight lens syndrome 11, 60, 66, 78, 105,
    132, 176
    lens removal 195
    plaque 80
    treatment 199
tinted, light-absorbing lenses 145
tonometry 117
trauma 5, 9, 186–7, 202
    blunt 186
    conjunctiva 34, 197
    consequences 188
    eyelid 196
treatment of complications 194–202
Tyndall phenomenon 59, 102, 116

uveitis 116, 121

viral infection 49, 52, 198
visual acuity 21
    impaired 35
    tight lens syndrome 78
visual impairment 120–1, 125–6
    deposits 151
    diagnostic evaluation 128
    intermittent 123
    permanent 121
    wetting problems 138

warm air provocation test 184
wearing time 3, 5, 60, 132, 139
welding 186
wetting agents 201
wetting problems 125–6, 138, 176
    deposits 151
wood splinters 186

Index to Illustrations

Note: numbers refer to figure numbers; those with suffix "*t*" refer to tables and those with suffix "*ill*" refer to illustrations within text

Acanthamoeba keratitis 258
adenovirus 13*t*
advantages of contact lenses over spectacles 3*t*
AIDS 52, 110, 256
allergy
  artificial tear solution 184
  chemosis 71, 72
  chlorhexidine 60, 74, 187
  eyelid 35–6, 39, 40, 43, 46, 49, 51–2, 54, 60, 71–2, 74, 76
  lens care products 193
  plant 76
  PMMA 194–5
  protein deposits 367
  quaternary ammonium bases 186
  thiomersal 41, 43, 50, 57, 74, 186, 187
aniridia, traumatic 17, 296
aphakia 10, 11, 17, 167, 251
  blepharoconjunctivitis 48
  conjunctival cyst 421
  dry eye 463
Aspergillus 13*t*, 303, 361
astigmatism 13, 15
  irregular 10, 267

bacterial infection 13*t*, 102–3, 106, 407
benzalkonium chloride 41, 43, 46, 72, 182, 198, 207
blepharitis 42, 50, 53
  squamous 37, 38, 51
blepharospasm 8*t*
break-up time (BUT) 448–51
bulb, perforated 17

CAB lens 66, 275, 306, 309
Candida 13*t*, 47, 109
cataract 12, 285
chalazion 392, 397
Chlamydia 13*t*
chlorbutanol 43
chlorhexidine 38, 41, 210
  allergic reaction 60, 74, 187
cleaning, faulty 342, 343, 346, 371
cobalt allergy 36, 54
complications, frequency 34*t*–37*t*
conjunctiva 55–9
  bulbar 73, 83, 116, 119
  chemosis 71, 72, 76
  compression 304, 307
  cutting injury 84
  cyst 395, 421–4
  edema 77, 94, 179
  fatty tissue prolapse 425
  foreign body reaction 46, 47
  hemorrhage 10*t*, 78, 81, 82, 85, 86, 87
  hyperemia 61–4, 88–92, 97, 102, 104–5, 112–15, 220, 229
    limbal 119, 121, 122, 223, 225
    perilimbal 113, 124, 212–13
    reactive 222
  injection 93, 95, 177, 312
    perilimbal 118, 221, 230
  injury 146
  irritation 96
  mechanical irritation 11*t*, 86, 88, 98

melanoma 420
melanosis 419
nevus 416–18
papilloma 413
phlyctena 409
swelling 212
tarsal 36, 64
tumor 414–15
vasodilatation 111, 116, 119, 222, 224
conjunctivitis 13*t*, 50
  bacterial 13*t*, 99–103, 106, 407
  chronic 302
  fungal 13*t*, 109, 110
  giant papillary 9*t*, 34, 63, 65–70
  mechanical irritation 220
  organisms 31*t*
  viral 13*t*, 107–8
contraindications for contact lenses 2
cornea
  abscess 257
  clouding 259
  cutting injury 83, 84
  cystic edema 172–4
  deformation 9*ill*
  endothelial changes 275–6, 276
  epithelial clouding 187, 189
  epithelial defect 254
  epithelial lesions 1*ill*, 2*ill*, 137, 138, 140–2, 145, 161, 163, 203–4
  erosion 30, 139, 141, 143, 147–50, 440–1
  fissures 130
  foreign body 2*ill*, 155, 224
  herpetic 164
  hypoxia 9*ill*, 168–71, 179, 221, 222, 237
  indentations 129
  infection 9*ill*
  infiltrates 134
  injury 9*ill*, 83, 84, 230
  lesion 156–60
  mechanical damage 203–4, 238
  metabolic decompensation 181
  metabolic impairment 10*ill*
  metabolic injury 230
  microtopography 7*ill*
  mosaic 132
  neovascularization 16*t*, 92, 94, 220–3, 241
  ophthalmometry 6*ill*
  pressure 4*ill*
  pseudoherpetic epithelial defect 161–3, 165
  pseudoinfiltrate 135–6
  scar 264–9, 271–4
  spiders 131, 185
  spiral traces 128
  staining 15*t*, 126
  stippling 127
  streaks 128
  stromal changes 168–9
  swelling coefficient 8*ill*
  tear 150, 156
  topography 277–84
  toric 293–4
  transplanted 241
  ulcers 17*t*, 101, 243–5, 247–56

faulty hygiene 300–1
  vascularization 213, 224, 226–8, 237–8, 254, 256, 268, 271–3
corneal deprivation syndrome 214–18
corneal distortion syndrome 283
corneal edema 15*t*, 81, 167–71, 176, 181, 183–6, 196, 201–4
  edge 142
  mixed solution syndrome 210–11
  neovascularization 229
  tear deficiency 442–3
  toxic keratopathy 236–7, 240
  toxic reactions 187–90, 192–5
corneal graft 347

dacrocystitis 405–6
deposits 348–51, 362–77
dermatitis, eyelid 36, 47, 49
diabetes mellitus 47, 109, 256–7
disadvantages of contact lenses compared with spectacles 4*t*
disinfection, thermal 219
displaced lens 297
disposable lenses 8, 12, 214–18
  breakage 338
  corneal epithelial defect 254
  corneal ulcer 250, 254
  edge defects 329
  fractures 322
  infection 242, 250
dry eye 426–32, 463
dystrichiasis 404

ectropion 403
eczema, eyelid 40, 41, 43
entropion 402
eye drops, abuse 75, 77
eyelid
  blepharitis 37–9
  cyst 396
  dermatitis 36, 47, 49
  diseases 391–403
  eczema 40, 41, 43
  hyperemia 60, 61
  papilloma 399
  tumour 398
  ulceration 54
  warts 401

febrile illness 249
fingernails 298
fitting 86
  poor 112–13
flour deposit 353
fluorosilicone carbonate lens 70
foreign body reaction 89, 92–4, 147, 155, 161, 347
  conjunctiva 89, 93
  corneal epithelial defect 2*ill*, 155
fungal infection 13*t*, 47, 109, 110

gel lens 7, 26
  chemosis 76
  conjunctival vasodilatation 116, 119
  conjunctivitis 100
  edge defects 81, 83

extended-wear 30
eyelid dermatitis 47
foreign body reaction 94
giant papillary conjunctivitis 69
hyperemia 234
irritation 96
mechanical/metabolic disturbance 225
mixed solution syndrome 212
tear deficiency 97
tight lens syndrome 178
tinted 29
toxic corneal injury 183–4, 186
toxic keratopathy 119
glare, causes 23*t*
glaucoma 10, 17

Haemophilus 13*t*, 48, 100
hairspray residue 354
handling, faulty 327, 330–2, 339
hard lens 1, 3, 4, 61
    broken edge 148
    CAB 5, 7
    chemosis 72
    conjunctival edema 77
    conjunctival hyperemia 113, 114
    conjunctival injury 146
    conjunctival vasodilatation 111
    conjunctivitis 107
    corneal cystic edema 174
    corneal edema 201–2
    corneal epithelial injury 142, 151, 152
    corneal erosion 143
    corneal hypoxia 168–9
    corneal scar 265–8, 274
    corneal ulcers 252
    corneal vascularization 231, 246
    defective 137, 141
    displaced to nasal canthus 289, 291
    dry eye 426–9, 432–3
    edge defects 82, 156
    faulty care 342, 346
    fitting error 306, 311, 313–14
    fluorosilicone carbonate 3
    foreign body reaction 89, 93, 155, 161
    improper insertion 139
    infection 244, 246
    mechanical irritation 58, 88
    opacification 337
    oxygen-permeable 5
    PMMA 1, 16, 44, 55, 68, 73, 175, 263, 270, 284
    scratches 317–21
    surface deposits 340
    tear deficiency 430, 452–5
herpes simplex virus 13*t*, 393, 394
hordeolum 391
hydrogen peroxide 159, 160, 188, 206, 209
hygiene, faulty 44, 159, 245, 362, 365–6
hyperopia 24
hypopyon 248
hyposphagma 80

immunocompromised patient 21*t*, 255
    see also AIDS; diabetes mellitus; leukemia
indications for contact lenses 1*t*
infection
    corneal 9*ill*
    diabetes mellitus 257
    disposable lenses 242
    eyelid 45–8, 50, 52

faulty hygiene 301
hard lens 244, 246
soft lens 243
    see also bacterial infection; conjunctivitis; fungal infection; viral infection
insertion of lens, improper 149–50, 152–3, 157
intraocular changes 20*t*
iris lens 296

Javal imaging 6*ill*
jelly-bump residue 349, 378–90

keratectomy, photoreflective 9
keratitis 135, 162, 164, 166, 248, 253
keratoconjunctivitis 3*ill*, 133
keratoconus 59, 262, 266, 274, 288, 292
keratopathy 134, 191, 205
    toxic 3*ill*, 87, 184, 186–7, 189, 198–9, 208–9
        corneal neovascularization 236
        corneal vascularization 232–4
        lens care products 236, 240
        mixed solution syndrome 213
        post-heat syndrome 219
        soft lens 120, 253
Klebsiella 13*t*

lacrimal pathway occlusion 405–6
lens care, faulty 342, 343, 346
lens care products 121, 197, 210
    allergy 53, 54, 193
    corneal epithelial defect 159, 160, 189
    toxic keratopathy 236, 240
    toxic reaction 182, 183, 186
lens case 300, 302–3
lens loss 286–7, 291
leukemia, corneal ulcer 255
leukoma, corneal 270

make-up 342, 345
manufacturing errors 338, 340
medication 38*t*
melanoma 420
melanosis 419
mercury allergy 36
metallic deposits 350, 352, 355–61
milium 400
mixed solution syndrome 210–13
Moraxella 13*t*
mucin deficiency 430, 433
myopia 14, 17, 19, 20, 22–3, 29, 32, 56, 313
    corneal pressure 5*ill*
    high 16, 247–8, 268, 270
    malignant 272

nevus 416–18
nickel allergy 36, 53

ocular disease 27*t*, 28*t*
ophthalmic preparations 38*t*
Ophthalmotest 3*ill*
orthokeratologic effect 280

panophthalmitis 257
patient education 5*t*
penicillin 51
phlyctena, conjunctival 409
piercing, intolerance to 53, 54
pinguecula 408

plano lens, tinted 28
PMMA allergy/intolerance 119, 123, 194–6, 234
PMMA lens 1*ill*, 85, 219, 263, 276
Pneumococcus 13*t*, 243, 249
Polyquad-II 199, 213
post-heat syndrome 219
preservative agents 54, 191, 205
pseudoepiscleritic irritation 125
pseudokeratitis 134, 260
pseudokeratoconus 9*ill*, 259, 284
Pseudomonas 13*t*, 101, 242, 245, 299, 301, 303
pseudopterygium 410–11
pseudoptosis 34
pterygium 412

quaternary ammonium bases 35, 71, 134, 186, 208

rigid gas-permeable (RGP) lens 19–21, 23, 32, 247, 277–83, 305
    cracks 341
    deposits 377
    trauma 465

sawdust deposit 351
sock phenomenon 372, 374
soft lens 13, 14, 25, 35
    Acanthamoeba keratitis 258
    AIDS 256
    cataract 285
    chemosis 71
    conjunctival hyperemia 115, 124, 229
    conjunctival perilimbal injection 118
    conjunctival vasodilatation 117
    conjunctivitis 108
    corneal cystic edema 172–3
    corneal defects 144, 154
    corneal fissures 130
    corneal hypoxia 170–1, 237
    corneal injury 238–9
    corneal neovascularization 220
    corneal scar 264, 269
    corneal transplant 241
    corneal ulcer 248–9, 251
    deposits 348–50, 353–5, 362, 366, 368–71, 373–5
    disposable 27
    dry eye 430
    edge defects 78, 84, 326, 328, 332, 334
    eye drop abuse 75
    eyelash trapped under 140
    faulty cleaning 343
    fitting error 304, 307–8, 310, 312, 315–16
    foreign body reaction 92, 147
    fracture 333, 336
    fungal infection 110
    giant papillary conjunctivitis 67
    hydrophilic 2, 31, 62
    improper insertion 139, 153
    infection 243
    jelly-bump residue 378–90
    keratitis 162, 248, 253, 256
    mechanical injury 261
    mechanical irritation 98
    metabolic disturbance 230
    metallic deposits 356–61
    PMMA 219, 310
    silicone 130, 135, 308, 312
    steeply fitted 222

tear 327
tear deficiency 434–6, 438–9, 457–62
toxic keratopathy 120, 253
trauma 464, 466
Staphylococcus 13*t*, 45, 52, 244, 250, 303
streptococcal infection 103
subconjunctival hemorrhage 10*t*, 43, 44
superinfection 45, 46, 48

tear deficiency 30*t*, 93, 96, 105, 111, 117,
    176, 426–9
aphakia 463
contraindication for lenses 456
corneal edema 442–3
corneal erosion 440–1

corneal metabolism impairment 10*ill*
hard lens 430, 452–5
jelly bumps 388
soft lens 434–6, 438–9, 457–62
tests 32*t*, 33*t*
tear film
break-up time (BUT) 448–51
instability 446–7
tear fluid actions 29*t*
tear lens 305, 313, 427, 429, 431
tear solution, artificial 72, 77, 184, 190
thiomersal, allergic reaction 74, 77, 104,
    124, 186–7, 192
tight lens syndrome 176–81
trauma 464

viral infection 13*t*, 107–8
visual impairment 22*t*, 24*t*, 25*t*

warts 401
wetting problem 426, 430, 435, 437, 443,
    444, 446